Green & Natural Antiviral Agents

Natural ways to prevent or treat viral infections

The recipes in this book contain easily obtained ingredients that are generally accepted to be safe and effective.

Individual reactions to the contained ingredients can vary. It is not possible to predict how any individual will react to a particular recipe, treatment, or ingredient.

As with any product, a user should employ common sense when creating these recipes or using the applicable ingredients. The reader should consult a qualified herbalist or physician before using any ingredient or recipe in this book.

The enclosed materials are for informational purposes only and the reader accepts all responsibility for determining the effectiveness and usefulness of all of the included items. Neither the author nor the publisher accepts and liability for the actions of the reader or for any reactions caused by the use of the contents and ingredients.

Nothing in this guide is intended to substitute for the medical expertise and advice of your primary health care provider.

You should discuss any decisions about treatment or care with your health care provider. The information contained within this guide is believed to be accurate at the time of writing but research is being undertaken daily and new information, effects, or side effects may be discovered that conflict with the materials contained herein.

No product, service, or therapy is endorsed by the author, publisher, or other individual associated with the creation of this material. The reader should remember that the U.S. Food and Drug Administration (FDA) have not evaluated the statements made in this book. The products listed are not intended to diagnose, treat, cure, or prevent any disease.

Using any medication whether prescription, over the counter, or herbal in nature may have a marked effect on your health and each medicine may interact with others. Tell your health care provider about any complementary, supplemental, or alternative practices you use including dietary substances, herbals, or oils.

Federal regulations for dietary supplements are different from the regulations applied to prescription and over the counter drugs. Dietary supplement manufacturers are not required to prove a product's safety and effectiveness.

Plant products are sometimes marketed as dietary supplements. Plant products do have a noticeable affect on the human body. The expected action of many plant products is based on traditional use and observation. Laboratory studies have been conducted to confirm the expected affect of some traditionally used plant products but others have not been researched in a laboratory setting. Most dietary supplements, herbs, and oils have not been researched for use by pregnant women, nursing women, or children. No supplement, herb, or oil in this book is recommended for use by women who are pregnant or nursing or by children.

Each person's needs and correct dosage will vary depending on a variety of factors. You should discuss your specific needs and best dosage with a qualified herbalist or physician.

Green & Natural Antiviral Agents

Natural ways to prevent or treat viral infections

Natural Antiviral & Immunostimulant Agents

The classification antiviral includes anything that destroys viruses or inhibits their ability to grow and reproduce.

Herbals approach viral infection from two directions. They stimulate the immune system to produce more immune cells aiding your body's ability to fight the infection and they act in direct opposition to viruses by inhibiting their ability to grow and reproduce so they cannot survive.

The first line of defense against viral infection is prevention . Disinfecting surfaces with known antiviral cleaners, maintaining good health through diet, rest, and exercise and minimizing exposure to infectious agents is far more effective than any treatment plan in the continued battle against viruses.

Regardless of the preventative care you take, there are always times where treating an infection will be necessary. Traditionally, viral infection is fought by blending herbals that support the body's own natural defenses with those that act to kill the virus. Using a combination that blends both actions helps to minimize the duration and severity of any infection.

Many herbs and oils act as natural immunostimulant and antiviral agents. Some of these natural products work as well as or even better than the products sold in your local pharmacy. Some of the items in your local pharmacy are even created based on the chemical constituents of plants you might have growing in your own yard.

This guide contains antiviral agents that act as both disinfectants for infected air and surfaces and disease fighting agents for the body. Both categories eliminate harmful viruses. It is important that you read the traditional uses and side effects of each plant and discuss any alternative treatment with a qualified herbalist or physician prior to choosing a natural product.

Ajwain, Ajava, Ajowan, Ajwon, Bishop's Flower, Bullwort, Caraway, Carom Seeds, Thymol Seeds

Botanical Names:
Trachyspermum ammi

Properties:
Abortifacient, Antibacterial, Antifungal, Anti-inflammatory, Antiseptic, Antispasmodic, Aphrodisiac, Aromatic, Bronchodilator, Digestive, Diaphoretic, Diuretic (roots), Expectorant, Hepatic, Relaxant, Vermifuge

Traditional Use:
Ajwain is traditionally used as a steam inhalant or essential oil aromatic to reduce the length and severity of the both bacterial and viral infections.

The high antibacterial, antifungal, and antiviral properties of Ajwain essential oil make it a traditional ingredient in air and spray based cleaning products.

Ajwain has long been a traditional treatment for infection and is undergoing research for its ability to combat drug resistant microbial pathogens.

Ajwain contains high levels of antifungal, antiviral, and antibacterial agents and is traditionally used to help enhance the immune system while combating infections.

Part Used:
Leaves, Seed, Oil

Side Effects:
Ajwain is not recommended for use by women who are pregnant or nursing. Ajwain has been used as an abortifacient in some cultures.

Ajwain is not recommended for use by diabetics due to the high sugar content.

Essential oils are for external use only and should be properly diluted prior to use.

Additional uses and side effects may exist but further research is necessary to determine the exact properties and effects of use.

General:
Ajwain is native to the Eastern Asia and Europe but has naturalized in many other regions where it has been harvested for hundreds of years for use as a spice or dried for use in traditional supplements. Ajwain is a frost tender annual that blooms from July to August. It is not particular regarding soil composition but does prefer full sun and consistent moisture. The seeds are harvested at the end of the flowering season and direct sown in the spring after all danger of frost has passed.

Ajwain seeds are used as a flavoring and it is cultivated as a spice product in some areas of the world. The seeds are harvested when ripe and distilled as an essential oil and the leaves, seeds, and oils are used as a traditional medicinal component and in perfumery.

Indian herbalists use the Ajwain leaf to create a strong decoction that is traditionally used at a rate of 2 teaspoons 2 times daily.

Aloe, Aloe Vera, Burn Plant, Elephant's Gall, Lily of the Desert, Sabila

Botanical Name:
Aloe vera, Aloe barbadensis

Properties:
Analgesic, Anti-inflammatory, Antibacterial, Antifungal, Emollient, Healing, Hypoallergenic, Hypoglycemic, Laxative

Traditional Use:
Aloe is traditionally used as a poultice for wound care because it is believed to have antibacterial, antifungal, and antiviral compounds that help to prevent wound infections.

Part Used:
Gel, Juice, Leaf

Side Effects:
Aloe bitters and aloe juice should not be taken internally during pregnancy, during menstruation, or in cases of rectal bleeding.

The laxative compounds in aloe are passed into mother's milk, so nursing mothers should avoid internal use of aloe.

Aloe can cause intense intestinal cramps if overused.

Overuse of aloe juice can cause diarrhea.

The FDA banned the use of aloe as a laxative ingredient in over-the-counter drug products in 2002, but it is widely used is commercial pharmaceuticals outside the United States.

The oral consumption of aloe leaf may cause cancer.

Consumption of aloe may cause lowered glucose levels.

Additional uses and side effects may exist but further research is necessary to determine the exact properties and effects of use.

General:
Aloe is succulent native to Africa but can be grown as a garden plant in other warm climates to zone 10 and is cultivated as an indoor plant worldwide. Aloe prefers moderately fertile, sandy soil with good drainage and full sunlight. Aloe is related to the cactus and each part of the plant contains substances that are used in supplement treatments.

The green part of the leaf that surrounds the gel is used to produce aloe juice or dried latex.

Andrographis, Indian Echinacea, Sambiloto

Botanical Name:
Andrographis paniculata

Properties:

Analgesic, Antibacterial, Antifungal, Anti-inflammatory, Antimicrobial, Antispasmodic, Antiviral, Astringent, Cholesterol, Febrifuge, Laxative, Immunostimulant, Sedative, Vermifuge

Traditional Use:
Recent studies indicate that Andrographis may help to stimulate the immune system and it has traditionally been used to lessen the frequency & severity of infections when ingested regularly as a tea or juice and immediately upon noticing the symptoms of an infection.

Andrographis has strong antibacterial and antiviral properties making it a traditional component in natural cleaning products.

Part Used:
Leaf, Juice

Side Effects:
Andrographis is not recommended for us by women who are pregnant or nursing.

Andrographis is not recommended for use by women or men who are attempting to conceive.

Andrographis is not recommended for use by people who have an autoimmune disease like Multiple Sclerosis or Lupus.

Overuse of Andrographis may cause serious allergic reactions.

Additional uses and side effects may exist but further research is necessary to determine the exact properties and effects of use.

General:
Andrographis is an herbaceous perennial native to Asia where it grows wild in the forests and wastelands. It can be cultivated elsewhere by direct or greenhouse sown seeds but needs 3-4 months of hot, humid weather to reach maturity.

The flower, leaf, and underground stem are harvested and juiced or dried for use in traditional supplement infusions sipped on an empty stomach.

Arborvitae, American Cedar, Emerald Green, Thuja, Tree of Life, White Cedar, Yellow Cedar

Botanical Name:
Thuja occidentalis

Properties:
Abortifacient, Antibacterial, Antifungal, Anti-inflammatory, Antiseptic, Antiviral, Arthritis, Astringent, Coagulant, Depurative, Diaphoretic, Diuretic, Emmenagogue, Expectorant, Immunostimulant, Nervine, Rubefacient, Sedative, Styptic, Vermifuge

Traditional Use:
Arborvitae leaves and twigs are used as a traditional supplement tea or extract for their stimulating, expectorant, and astringent properties. They are used as a traditional treatment for respiratory problems like asthma, bronchitis, colds, congestion, influenza, and pneumonia. Arborvitae is traditionally used to help stimulate antibodies and shorten the intensity and duration of bacterial and viral conditions.

Arborvitae is used as a traditional supplement to boost the immune system and to help increase antibody production in the body and fight infections such as colds, herpes, HIV, influenza, and other infections.

Part Used:
Green Branches / Twigs, Leaf - Oil

Side Effects:
Arborvitae is a known abortifacient and should not be used by women who are pregnant or nursing.

Arborvitae has been used as an abortifacient in some cultures.

Arborvitae oil is toxic and should not be taken internally for extended periods.

Arborvitae oil should only be used under the care of a qualified herbalist or physician.

Arborvitae oil is a neurotoxin and use may cause convulsions, diarrhea, gastro-enteritis, increased heart rate, and spasms in high doses.

Arborvitae has immunostimulant properties and should not be used by individuals who have an immunoreactive illness like Multiple Sclerosis and Lupus.

Additional uses and side effects may exist but further research is necessary to determine the exact properties and effects of use.

General:
Arborvitae is an evergreen shrub native to North America and Asia that grows easily and is adapted to a variety of soil, sun, and water conditions though it prefers humid weather and regular watering. Arborvitae is propagated by seeds sown out as soon as they are ripe or by cuttings taken in the late summer.

Arborvitae wood is used in crafts, fence posts, and shingle making. The oils of the Arborvitae have been used as cleaners and insecticides. The foliage is used as a source of vitamin C. The shoot pith is eaten as a cooked vegetable or added to stews. The inner bark is cooked and eaten or dried and ground to flour.

Arborvitae is typically harvested in the spring when the oil is extracted by steam distillation and the leaves & twigs are dried, powdered, and incorporated into traditional supplement infusions. 1 teaspoon of the leaves and tops were boiled in 2 cups of water by the Native Americans who then administered 1 tablespoon at a time to alleviate most internal symptoms or the oils were incorporated into recipes for topical preparations.

Arrowleaf, Balsamroot, Oregon Sunflower

Botanical Name: Balsamorhiza sagittata

Properties: Antibacterial, Antiseptic, Cathartic, Diaphoretic, Diuretic, Expectorant, Febrifuge, Immunostimulant, Sedative, Stimulant, Vulnerary

Traditional Use: Arrowleaf root is believed to strengthen the immune system in a manner similar to Echinacea and is used in traditional preparations at a rate of 1-teaspoon tincture 2 times a day.

Arrowleaf root, stem, and leaf infusions have traditionally been used to reduce fever, expel excess mucus and increase immunity in common infections like bronchitis, colds, and influenza while acting to reduce the severity and duration of the underlying infection.

Part Used: Root

Side Effects: Arrowleaf is not recommended for use by women who are pregnant or nursing.

Arrowleaf may cause an allergic reaction in some people.

Additional uses and side effects may exist but further research is necessary to determine the exact properties and effects of use.

General: Arrowleaf is native to much of Western North America and is able to adapt to a variety of environmental conditions from desert to grassland to forest. A member of the sunflower family, it prefers moist soil and full sun and is propagated by seed but does not transplant well.

Arrowleaf roots, young shoots, and seeds have been eaten as a raw or cooked vegetable. The seeds are ground for a highly nutritious flour product and the leaves are boiled and eaten. The seeds yield a rich oil and the root has been roasted and ground as a coffee substitute.

Arrowleaf roots have been harvested for use as a traditional supplement for hundreds of years. The most common use for Arrowleaf is as an immunostimulant traditionally given as 1 teaspoon of the root tincture twice daily.

Astragalus, Bei Qu, Huang Qi, Milk Vetch, Mongolian Milk, Ogi

Botanical Name:
Astragalus membranaceus

Properties:
Adaptogen, Antibacterial, Antihistamine, Anti-inflammatory, Antiviral, Cancer, Cardiotonic, Diuretic, Febrifuge, Hypoglycemic, Hypotensive, Immunostimulant, Nervine, Stimulant, Vasodilator

Traditional Use:
Astragalus capsules or teas are traditionally taken as an immunostimulant and preventative.

Astragalus contains bioflavonoid, choline, and polysaccharide that have traditionally been used to strengthen the immune system and act as a preventative against bacterial & viral infections.

Astragalus has traditionally been used as part of a regimen geared toward helping to restore immune function in compromised individuals.

Part Used:
Root

Side Effects:
Astragalus is not recommended for use by women who are pregnant or nursing.

Astragalus may increase bleeding.

Astragalus may interfere with the effectiveness of a class of high blood pressure medications known as beta-blockers and with drugs that suppress the immune system.

Astragalus may affect blood sugar levels and blood pressure.

Caution should be used if you are on an immunosuppressive therapy as Astragalus may have immunostimulant properties.

Additional uses and side effects may exist but further research is necessary to determine the exact properties and effects of use.

General:
Astragalus is native to China but can be cultivated in full sun, sandy and well-drained soil in other regions. Growing up to 6 feet tall, Astragalus is hardy to zone 6. It flowers in the late summer with the seeds ripening as the blooms pass their peak. Astragalus is difficult to propagate, as seed germination tends to be erratic. The seeds should be harvested when they are fresh, soaked, and then planted out immediately.

The roots of mature plants are harvested and incorporated into soups and teas or ingested as a tincture or powder capsule traditionally given at a rate of up to 5 tablespoons of the dried herb daily.

Autumn Olive, Autumn Berry, Japanese Silverberry

Botanical Name: Elaeagnus umbellata

Properties: Antibacterial, Astringent, Cancer, Cardiotonic, Stimulant

Traditional Use: The flowers are used as a traditional supplement to ease constriction of bronchial passages and stimulate mucus-producing coughs in conditions like asthma, bronchitis, colds, and influenza while acting to stimulate the immune system and minimize the duration of infections.

Side Effects: Autumn Olive is not recommended for use by women who are pregnant or nursing.

Autumn Olive flowers are believed to be a cardiac stimulant and should not be used without the advice of a physician or qualified herbalist.

Additional uses and side effects may exist but further research is necessary to determine the exact properties and effects of use.

General: Autumn Olive is deciduous shrub common in thin woods and lowland areas of Asia. It has been naturalized in other regions of the world where it is easily propagated by seed. Autumn Olive is hardy to zone 3 and is considered an invasive species in some parts of the Eastern United States. The Autumn Olive is often propagated by seed but may take two years to germinate. It can also be propagated by air layering or cuttings of branches taken in mid-summer. Autumn Olive is cultivated for its ability to fix nitrogen into poor quality or exhausted soils.

The fruit is eaten raw or cooked and is a source of essential fatty acids. The flowers, leaves, and seed are harvested for use in traditional supplements

Bailahuen

Botanical Name: Haplopappus baylahuen

Properties: Antiinflammatory, Antioxidant, Astringent, Diaphoretic, Stimulant

Traditional Use: Bailahuen oils are traditionally used in aromatherapy treatments to minimize the congestive symptoms of an upper respiratory tract infection like bronchitis, colds, and influenza and to help to stimulate the immune system helping to shorten the duration and severity of common viral infections.

Part Used: Resin, Oil

Side Effects: Bailahuen is not recommended for use by women who are pregnant or nursing.

Bailahuen may cause an allergic reaction in some people.

Additional uses and side effects may exist but further research is necessary to determine the exact properties and effects of use.

General:
Bailahuen is shrub native to Chile and cultivated in other regions. Hardy to zone 9, it prefers well-drained soil and full sun. It is propagated by seeds sown out as soon as they are ripe.

Bailahuen resin has been harvested for use in traditional supplements for hundreds of years. Bailahuen has recently been discovered to have antioxidant properties and is being researched to determine what other potential benefits and side effects it might offer.

Balsam of Peru, Tolu, Quina

Botanical Name: Myroxylon pereirae

Properties: Antibacterial, Anti-inflammatory, Antifungal, Antiseptic, Antiviral, Aromatic, Stimulant

Traditional Use: Balsam of Peru oils are traditionally used to treat fungal, parasitic, and viral skin related infections including conditions like athlete's foot, staphylococcus, scabies, and lice.

Part Used: Bark Resin

Side Effects: Balsam of Peru is not recommended for use by women who are pregnant or nursing.

Balsam of Peru may be absorbed through the skin and prolonged or extensive use may cause kidney damage.

Balsam of Peru may cause allergic reactions in some people.

Balsam of Peru may cause sensitivity to sunlight.

Additional uses and side effects may exist but further research is necessary to determine the exact properties and effects of use.

General: Balsam of Peru is indigenous to the tropical forests of South America but is cultivated elsewhere for its wood and perfumery uses. It is mainly propagated by suckering but can also be propagated by seed and will self-propagate easily in a variety of soil, sun, and moisture conditions. It is considered an invasive species in some tropical regions.

The wood is sometimes used in woodcraft and the resin is frequently used in perfumery or as a flavoring. The oily resin is harvested for use in traditional topical preparations at a rate of 10% total volume, personal care products, and as a fragrance in perfumes, feminine care products, and household cleaners.

Baobab, Adansonia, Boabab, Cream of Tarter Tree, Boki, Senegal, Upside Down Tree

Botanical Name: Adansonia digitata

Properties: Antiinflammatory, Antiasthmatic, Antioxidant, Astringent, Diaphoretic, Expectorant, Emollient, Febrifuge, Immuno-Stimulant

Traditional Use: Baobab is traditionally given as a 5-gram daily supplement to help stimulate the immune system and promote resistance to common viral infections.

Part Used: Bark, Fruit, Leaf, Seed - Oil

Side Effects: Baobab is not recommended for use by women who are pregnant or nursing.

Additional uses and side effects may exist but further research is necessary to determine the exact properties and effects of use.

General: Baobab is a tree native to Africa and naturalized to most tropical countries. Baobab is easily propagated by seed preferring full sunlight and moist soil though it is drought tolerant once established. The Baobab tree docs not tolerate cold but can be grown in containers in colder regions.

Baobab is harvested as a food for the indigenous peoples of Africa. It has a unique nutritional content and is considered by some to be the next likely super food. Baobab oils are extracted by cold pressing the seeds and the bark and leaves are harvested, dried, and powdered for use in traditional supplement preparations.

Beggars Tick, Beggar Tick, Beggers Tick, Spanish Needles

Botanical Name: Bidens frondosa

Properties: Antiinflammatory, Antiviral, Astringent, Diuretic, Expectorant, Stimulant

Traditional Use: Beggars Tick seeds are used in a traditional infusion to help expel excess mucus associated with congestive conditions like asthma, bronchitis, colds, and influenza while acting to reduce the duration and severity of any related infection.

Part Used: Root, Seed

Side Effects: Beggers Tick is not recommended for use by women who are pregnant or nursing.

Beggars Tick may cause an allergic reaction or skin irritation in some people.

Additional uses and side effects may exist but further research is necessary to determine the exact properties and effects of use.

General:
Beggars Tick is native to North America where it can be found growing along ditches, ponds, and untended moist areas. It is not particular regarding soil composition but requires full sun and regular moisture. Beggers Tick can be propagated by seeds sown out after all danger of frost has passed.

The young leaves and stems are eaten as a cooked vegetable. The roots and seeds are harvested for use in traditional supplement infusions.

Bergamot, Beebalm, Fragrant Balm, High Balm, Indian Plume, Mountain Balm

Botanical Name: Monarda didyma

Properties: Analgesic, Antibacterial, Antifungal, Antiviral, Antispasmodic, Digestive, Nervine, Sedative

Traditional Use: Bergamot is an antibacterial, antiviral, analgesic and has been used in traditional treatments.

Bergamot essential oil is traditionally used against a variety of microorganisms and is often included as part of natural antibacterial and antiviral cleaning agents.

Bergamot is used in traditional topical preparations, gargles, and infusions to alleviate canker sores and to reduce the number and severity of herpes simplex outbreaks.

Bergamot has been used in traditional gargle treatments to ease a sore throat and combat infection in the throat and mouth by blending 3 drops of bergamot oil in ½-cup warm water with ¼-teaspoon salt.

Part Used: Fruit, Leaf, Peel Oil

Side Effects: Bergamot is not recommended for use by women who are pregnant or nursing.

Bergamot is not recommended for use in children's treatments.

Bergamot increases sun sensitivity. Do not use on the skin when sun exposure is likely.

Additional uses and side effects may exist but further research is necessary to determine the exact properties and effects of use.

General: Bergamot is native to Asia and Eastern North America. Hardy to zone 4, it is not particular regarding soil composition but does prefer steady moisture and full to partial sun. Bergamot is propagated by seed planted in the late spring or by division in the spring or fall.

Bergamot leaves and young shoots are eaten as a raw or cooked vegetable. Bergamot fruit and leaves are harvested for use in topical &

internal preparations as well as in fragrances, inhalant therapy, and natural care products.

Birthwort, Guang Fang Ji, Pelican Flower, Pipevines, Red River Snakeroot, Sangree Root, Sangrel, Snakeroot, Snakeweed, Virginia Serpentary

Botanical Name:
Aristolochia clematitis

Properties:
Abortifacient, Antibacterial, Anti-inflammatory, Antispasmodic, Antiviral, Cancer, Depurative, Diaphoretic, Emmenagogue, Febrifuge, Immunostimulant, Nervine

Traditional Use:
Birthwort has shown some ability to stimulate the immune system and is used in traditional immunity building regimen.

Birthwort is traditionally used in washes to fight herpes simplex infections of the eye.

Birthwort has shown some ability to promote antibacterial and antiviral effects in the body and has traditionally been used to treat a wide array of infections.

Birthwort has been used in traditional topical preparations to cleanse, prevent infection, and speed healing in skin sores, ulcers, and wounds.

Part Used:
Blooming Flower, Root

Side Effects:
Birthwort is not recommended for use by women who are pregnant or nursing.

Birthwort has been used as an abortifacient in some cultures.

Birthwort contains aristolochic acid that is considered toxic and has been banned for use in many parts of the world.

Birthwort can cause nausea, abdominal pain, and vomiting.

Overuse of birthwort is toxic and can cause gastrointestinal upset, kidney damage, respiratory paralysis, spasms, vomiting, and even death.

Do not use birthwort until you have consulted a qualified herbalist or physician to determine if there is a less dangerous and more effective treatment available for your particular needs.

Additional uses and side effects may exist but further research is necessary to determine the exact properties and effects of use.

General:
Birthwort is native to Europe, North America, and Mexico but has been naturalized to other parts of the world and is considered an invasive weed by some. Hardy to zone 6, it prefers rich, shady woods for growth but will grow in any soil composition or sun situation. Birthwort can be propagated by seed sown as soon as they are ripe in the fall, division in the fall, or by root cuttings taken in the late winter.

Birthwort was once a commonly used supplement treatment for a variety of body systems but has fallen out of preference due to the potential for toxicity. If Birthwort is indicated for a particular disorder, the advice of a qualified herbalist or physician should be sought.

Biscuit Root, Fernleaf Biscuit Root

Botanical Name:
Lomatium dissectum

Properties:
Antibacterial, Antiviral, Antimicrobial, Expectorant, Immunostimulant, Ophthalmic, Stimulant

Traditional Use:

Biscuit Root is a stimulating expectorant traditionally burnt and inhaled, included in steam baths, or given as a supplement to alleviate congestion in conditions like asthma, bronchitis, colds, influenza, and pneumonia while acting so treat any underlying infection and shorten the duration of the illness.

Biscuit Root has both antibacterial and antiviral properties making it a common traditional supplement or topical preparation to help treat bacterial and viral infections.

Biscuit Root is commonly used in traditional disinfectant cleansers and as a steam air purifier.

Biscuit Root is used as a traditional preparation to stimulate the immune system helping to prevent or shorten the duration and severity of infections.

Part Used:
Resin, Root

Side Effects:
Biscuit Root is not recommended for use by women who are pregnant or nursing.

Biscuit Root is not recommended for use by people with an immunoreactive disorder like Multiple Sclerosis or Lupus.

Biscuit Root may cause an allergic reaction or a full body skin rash in some people.

Additional uses and side effects may exist but further research is necessary to determine the exact properties and effects of use.

General:
Biscuit Root is a flowering plant native to western North America and adaptable to a wide range of soil and water conditions. It does require full sun. Biscuit Root is propagated by seed sown as soon as it is ripe and self-seeds readily.

The root is eaten as a cooked vegetable or dried and ground for use as a thickening agent or flour additive.   The root and resin have been harvested for hundreds of years for use in supplement preparations to alleviate a variety of infectious conditions.

Bitter Damson, Dysentery Bark, Mountain Damson, Simarouba, Slave Wood, Stave Wood

Botanical Name:
Simarouba amara

Properties:
Abortifacient, Analgesic, Antibacterial, Antiviral, Astringent, Cancer, Diuretic, Febrifuge, Immunostimulant, Tonic, Vermifuge

Traditional Uses:
Bitter Damson has been used as a traditional supplement to stimulate the immune system acting to prevent infection or shorten the duration of infection when taken as soon as systems appear.

Bitter Damson is traditionally used to treat both bacterial and viral infections.

Parts Used:
Bark

Side Effects:
Bitter Damson is not recommended for use by women who are pregnant or nursing.

Bitter Damson has been used as an abortifacient.

Overuse of Bitter Damson may cause gastrointestinal upset.

Additional uses and side effects may exist but further research is necessary to determine the exact properties and effects of use.

General:

Bitter Damson is a tree native to the Caribbean and South America but has been cultivated in other regions. It is not particular regarding soil composition but requires full sun and high moisture.

Bitter Damson is used in woodcraft and papermaking but is most valued as a veneer product. The wood requires pest protection treatment. The bark is harvested, dried, and powdered for use in traditional supplements. Bitter Damson has recently gained interest by researches for its potential in treating viral infections, stimulating the immune system, and preventing or treating cancer.

Bitter Melon, African Cucumber, Ampalaya, Balsam Pear, Blasamine, Bitter Gourd, Carella Fruit, Cerasee, Goya, Wild Cucumber

Botanical Name:
Momordica charantia

Properties:
Abortifacient, Antioxidant, Antiviral, Astringent, Cancer, Cardiac, Contraceptive, Hypoglycemic, Immunostimulant, Stimulant

Traditional Use:
Bitter melon has shown immunostimulant properties that make it a traditional component in preventing or shortening the duration of certain types of infections including colds, influenza, and other viruses

Bitter Melon is used as a traditional treatment to kill both non-drug resistant and drug resistant viruses including herpes.

Bitter melon has traditionally been used as a treatment of infections caused by retroviruses, colds, influenza, and other viral infections.

Part Used:
Whole Fruit

Side Effects:
Bitter Melon is not recommended for use by women who are pregnant or nursing.

Bitter Melon is known to have abortifacient properties.

Do not use bitter melon if you are planning to become pregnant as bitter melon has a documented ability to reduce fertility in both men and women.

Bitter melon affects the body's blood sugar levels and you should consult a physician prior to implementing a treatment plan based on bitter melon.

Additional uses and side effects may exist but further research is necessary to determine the exact properties and effects of use.

General:
Bitter melon is a climbing vine reaching 6 feet in height and native to southern Asia. It has been cultivated in some warmer regions as an ornamental of for the edible fruits.   Bitter Melon is propagated by seed and prefers full sun, consistent moisture, and well-drained loamy soil.

Bitter melon fruits are harvested while young and cooked as a food or used to make a beer like product. Bitter melon fruit is often added as a dietary supplement, the fruit juices are traditionally given as a supplement, and the dried melon is used as a supplement tea.

Black Alder, Alder, Smooth Alder, Tag Alder

Botanical Name: Alnus glutinosa

Properties: Antiparasitic, Antiviral, Astringent, Cathartic, Colorant, Dental, Emetic, Febrifuge, Galacogogue, Insecticide, Purgative, Styptic, Tonic, Vermifuge

Traditional Use: Black Alder bark decoctions have been used as a traditional topical preparation to reduce inflammation, treat infection, and speed healing in skin condtions like contact dermatitis, persistent sores, ulcers, and wounds.

Black Alder leaves and dried bark are traditionally powdered for use as a gargle to treat throat pain and inflammation and has shown some ability to clear staph and strep infections.

Part Used: Bark, Leaves

Side Effects: Black Alder is not recommended for use by women who are pregnant or nursing.

Black Alder bark is purgative when fresh. Only dried and powdered bark is used in supplement preparations.

Additional uses and side effects may exist but further research is necessary to determine the exact properties and effects of use.

General:
Black Alder is native to Asia, Europe, and North America. Hardy to zone 3, it prefers loamy or clay soil, full or partial sun, and moist to wet conditions. Black Alder grows quickly and has a reputation for fixing nitrogen into poor quality soil. Black Alder is cultivated by seeds sown as soon as they are ripe or by cuttings taken in the late fall and planted in sandy soil throughout the winter.

Black Alder is prized for yielding a wide range of dye products. The bark of the Black Alder yields a red toned dye used as a textile colorant and to make ink. The buds yield a green toned dye. Fresh, green Black Alder wood yields a fawn colored dye product. The bark and young shoots yield a yellow toned dye. Shoots harvested as soon as they appear yield a dusky brown toned colorant. The fruits yield a dark red toned dye.

Black Alder wood is water durable and has been used in a variety of maritime woodcraft.

Black Alder bark and leaves are harvested in the spring, dried and powdered for use in traditional supplements made with 1 teaspoon powder in 1 cup liquid. Fresh bark is purgative so only the dried bark is traditionally used for most treatments.

Black Cherry, Black Choke, Chokecherry, Rum Cherry, Virginian Prune, Wild Cherry

Botanical Name:
Prunus serotina

Properties:
Anodyne, Antibacterial, Anti-inflammatory, Antitussive, Antiviral, Astringent, Colorant, Expectorant, Sedative, Tonic

Traditional Use:
Black Cherry bark and fruits are a traditional tincture cough remedy and is a primary component in many commercial cough treatments. Black cherry contains compounds that are excreted through the lungs increasing respiration and sedating the nerves that provoke a cough reflex that combines well with the antibacterial and antiviral effect to make it a treatment in asthma, bronchitis, colds, congestion, non-productive coughs, influenza, pneumonia, and whooping cough.

Black Cherry is antiviral & antibacterial and is traditionally used to minimize the length and severity of infections including upper respiratory infections like the common cold, bacterial pneumonia, and influenza.

Part Used:
Bark, Fruit

Side Effects:
Black Cherry is not recommended for use by women who are pregnant or nursing.

Black Cherry is not for long-term use.

Black Cherry bark contains a highly poisonous substance called prussic acid and overuse can be toxic.

Additional uses and side effects may exist but further research is necessary to determine the exact properties and effects of use.

General:

Black Cherry is deciduous tree native to North America and cultivated in Europe. Hardy to zone 3, it is not particular regarding soil composition but requires full sun and consistent moisture. It can be propagated by seed sown out as soon as it is ripe, by air layering in the spring, or by cuttings taken between spring and mid summer.

Black Cherry leaves yield a green toned dye product and the fruit yields a grayish green colorant. The wood is valued in woodcraft and the fruit is eaten raw or cooked in jams, preserves, and pastry. The juices of the fruit have also been used as a food, beverage, or medicinal flavoring. A decoction of the bark is used as a flavoring in baked goods, beverages, and medicinals while the young twigs are used as a hot or cold beverage.

Black Cherry bark and fruits are harvested for use in commercial and traditional supplement syrups. The bark separates from the tree easily making it easy to harvest, dry and power for use in traditional supplement tinctures, syrups, or infusions. It should not be boiled since this may destroy some of the active components so it is traditionally administered at a rate of 1-teaspoon bark steeped in 1-cup warm water given in 2 teaspoonful doses up to 3 times a day.

Black Currant, Cassis

Botanical Name: Ribes nigrum

Properties: Antiinflammatory, Antimicrobial, Astringent, Cholesterol, Colorant, Diaphoretic, Diuretic, Febrifuge, Immuno-Stimulant

Traditional Uses: Black Currents contain high levels of GLA and is used as a traditional supplement to help stimulate the immune system and ward off or shorten the duration and severity of infections.

Black Current leaf has traditionally been used as a gargle to help speed the healing of mouth ulcers and to alleviate the associated infection, pain & inflammation in both the sores and in sore throats.

Black Current has been used as a traditional wash to help prevent infection and speed the healing of wounds and skin ulcers.

Parts Used: Fruit, Leaf, Seed – Oil

Side Effects: Black Currant is not recommended for use by women who are pregnant or nursing.

Black current may slow blood clotting.

Additional uses and side effects may exist but further research is necessary to determine the exact properties and effects of use.

General:
Black Current is a berry native to Asia and Europe but cultivated in many other regions. Hardy to zone 5, it is not particular regarding soil composition but does prefer good drainage, consistent moisture, and full or partial sun. It is propagated by seed planted out in the fall as soon as they are ripe or by cuttings taken in the late summer or early winter with a heel of old growth.

The fruits yield a blue or light purple dye product and are eaten raw or cooked as a food or drink component. The leaves are used as a soup seasoning or tea substutite and the seed oil is valued for natural skin care preparations. The leaves are harvested for use fresh or dried in traditional topical and tea supplements.

Black Locust

Botanical Name:
Robinia pseudoacacia

Properties:
Analgesic, Antispasmodic, Antiviral, Cancer, Chalagogue, Colorant, Diuretic, Emetic, Emollient, Expectorant, Febrifuge, Laxative, Narcotic

Traditional Use:
Black Locust leaves are used as a traditional tea or cleaning component to inhibit the spread of viral infections like colds and influenza.

Part Used:
Flower, Leaf, Seed

Side Effects:
Black Locust is not recommended for use by women who are pregnant or nursing.

The seed of the Black Locust may have narcotic properties and while the leaf has been shown to have antiviral properties, it may be purgative.

Black Locust may cause an allergic reaction in some people.

Additional uses and side effects may exist but further research is necessary to determine the exact properties and effects of use.

General:
Black Locust is native to the eastern North America and naturalized in areas of Africa, Asia, and Europe. Hardy to zone 3, it is not particular regarding soil composition and will grow in nutritionally poor soils. It requires full sun and dry to lightly moist soil. Black Locust can be propagated by seeds soaked in water and then sown in the early spring. Suckers can be divided from the mother plant during the dormant season.

The bark yields a yellow toned dye product that can be used with a variety of different mordants to achieve different shading. The seeds are boiled in the pod and eaten as a cooked pea-like vegetable. The fruits are skinned and the skins used to make a narcotic beverage.   The wood is harvested for use in crafting, general construction and for other purposes where a strong, durable wood is needed. The essential oils from the flowers are used in perfumery.

The seeds are cooked and eaten as a food or ground into flour for use in baking or cooking. The flowers are dried and powdered for supplement infusions and food purposes.

Bladderwrack, Atlantic Kelp, Black Tang, Bladder Fucus, Cutweed, Fucus, Kelp, Kelpware, Knotted Wrack, Marine Oak, Norwegian Seaweed, Marina

Rockweed, Rockweed, Rockwrack, Sea Kelp, Seaweed, Seawrack, Tang, Varech

Botanical Name:
Fucus vesiculosus

Properties:
Analgesic, Antibacterial, Antiviral, Anti-inflammatory, Appetite Suppressant, Contraceptive, Laxative, Hyperthyroid, Hypoglycemic, Laxative

Traditional Use:
Bladderwrack has shown some level of antiviral and antibacterial ability and has traditionally been used to inhibit bacterial infections and viruses.

Part Used:
Whole

Side Effects:
Bladderwrack is not recommended for use by women who are pregnant or nursing.

Bladderwrack is not recommended for use by individuals attempting to conceive as it may lower fertility.

Bladderwrack is a thyroid stimulant and is not recommended for use by people who have a thyroid condition or are on medication affecting the thyroid without the guidance of a qualified physician or herbalist.

Bladderwrack contains high amounts of iodine and may affect the thyroid in individuals who do not have a previous thyroid disorder and may raise the risk of thyroid cancer.

Bladderwrack may cause an allergic reaction in some people.

Additional uses and side effects may exist but further research is necessary to determine the exact properties and effects of use.

General:

Bladderwrack is seaweed found growing on the coasts of the northern water bodies including the Atlantic Ocean, Baltic Sea, Pacific Ocean, and the North Sea. It is harvested year round along both the east and west coastline of North America and other countries and used at a 1:1 dilution in extracts for supplement use with the traditional dosage being 1 teaspoon administered 3 times daily.

Blue Green Algae, Cyanbacteria, Hawaiian Spirulina, Lake Algae, Spirulina

Botanical Name:
Arthrospira platensis

Properties:
Antihistamine, Antioxidant, Antiviral, Cancer, Immunostimulant

Traditional Use:
Blue Green Algae is used in traditional supplements to prevent certain types of infections and prevent or treat cancer. Studies indicate that Blue Green Algae boosts immune system function. The research into the potential benefits to the immune system is ongoing.

A compound isolated in Blue Green Algae has shown some ability in laboratory studies to inhibit the cytomegalovirus, herpes simplex virus, measles, and mumps.

Part Used:
Whole Dried Algae- Powder

Side Effects:
Blue Green Algae is not recommended for use by women who are pregnant or nursing.

Blue Green Algae is not recommended for use in children's treatments.

Caution should be taken to ensure that the source of the Blue Green Algae is not contaminated through groundwater, bacteria, or another source.

Blue Green Algae is believed to stimulate the immune system and is not recommended for use by individuals who have an immunity related disorder like Multiple Sclerosis or Lupus.

Additional uses and side effects may exist but further research is necessary to determine the exact properties and effects of use.

General:
Blue Green Algae thrives in warm, fresh water lakes and is found in abundance in inland bodies of water that are both warm and alkaline but it can be cultivated, harvested, dried, and powdered for use in supplements and has traditionally been used at a rate between 250 milligrams to 5 grams daily.

Boxwood, Boj, Bush Tree

Botanical Name:
Buxus sempervirens

Properties:
Antiviral, Astringent, Cathartic, Cholagogue, Colorant, Diaphoretic, Febrifuge, Immunostimulant, Sedative, Vermifuge

Traditional Use:
Boxwood leaf extract is traditionally used to stimulate the immune system helping to ward off and treat viral infections.

Boxwood extract has shown an ability to help stop viruses from reproducing and is used in antiviral supplement and cleaning preparations.

Boxwood has been used in traditional supplements to help delay the progression of HIV – AIDS and additional research is being conducted to determine the properties, side effects, and potential of Boxwood extracts.

Part Used:
Leaf

Side Effects:

Boxwood is not recommended for use by women who are pregnant or nursing.

Only leaf extracts are used in supplement preparations as the whole, fresh leaf may have serious side effects like paralysis, seizures, and even death.

Boxwood bark has known sedative properties and is not recommended for use without the guidance of a qualified herbalist or physician.

Boxwood leaf is not recommended for internal use without the guidance of a qualified herbalist or physician.

Additional uses and side effects may exist but further research is necessary to determine the exact properties and effects of use.

General:
Boxwood is native to Europe but has been naturalized to many other parts of the world where it is cultivated as an ornamental. Hardy to zone 5, it is not particular regarding soil composition but does prefer full to partial sun and dry to moist soil. Boxwood can be propagated by seed, spring cuttings, or air layering.

Boxwood is commonly used as a designed or privacy hedge and the leaves yield a burgundy color dye product used in textile and hair coloring agents. Boxwood leaves are harvested in the spring and the dried leaf or leaf extracts are used in traditional topical and supplemental preparations.

Brown Kelp, Alginate, Giant Kelp, Pacific Kelp, Sea Kelp, Sea Whistle

Botanical Name:
Macrocystis pyrifera

Properties:
Antiviral, Cholesterol, Hypotensive, Immunostimulant

Traditional Use:

Brown Kelp has been shown to have antiviral qualities and is traditionally used to help stimulate the immune system and ward off viruses including influenza.

Part Used:
Whole

Side Effects:
Brown kelp is not recommended for use by women who are pregnant or nursing.

Brown kelp is a source of iodine and should not be used by those who have hyperthyroidism.

Additional uses and side effects may exist but further research is necessary to determine the exact properties and effects of use.

General:
Brown Kelp is found primarily along the western coast of North America. It is harvested for use as a binding agent and in traditional supplements.

Bupleurum, Bei Chai Hu, Hare's Ear, Sickle Leaf, Thoroughwax

Botanical Name:
Bupleurum falcatum

Properties:
Analgesic, Antibacterial, Anti-inflammatory, Antitussive, Antiviral, Carminative, Diaphoretic, Emmenagogue, Febrifuge, Hepatic, Immunostimulant, Sedative

Traditional Use:
Bupleurum has been used in traditional supplements to help reduce the fever and cough associated with conditions like bronchitis, colds, influenza, and pneumonia and to help reduce the length and severity of the infection.

Bupleurum has traditionally been used in supplements to minimize the number and severity of herpes simplex outbreaks.

Part Used:
Root

Side Effects:
Bupleurum is not recommended for use by women who are pregnant or nursing.

Bupleurum is not recommended for use by people with an autoimmune disorder like Multiple Sclerosis or Lupus.

Bupleurum is not recommended for use by people who are undergoing treatment for hepatitis or are taking antibiotics.

Additional uses and side effects may exist but further research is necessary to determine the exact properties and effects of use.

General:
Bupleurum is native to Asia and Europe but is cultivated in other regions. Hardy to zone 3, it is not particular regarding soil composition but does prefer full to partial sun and dry to moist soil. Bupleurum can be propagated by seed sown out in the spring or by division of the clumps.

The root, leaves, and young shoots are eaten as a cooked vegetable and the root has been harvested, dried, and powdered for thousands of years for use in traditional supplements.

Cajeput, Paperbark Tree, Swamp Tea Tree, White Tea Tree

Botanical Name:
Melaleuca leucadendron

Properties:
Analgesic, Antibacterial, Antimicrobial, Antiviral, Astringent, Carminative, Emollient, Estrogenic, Expectorant, Febrifuge, Immunostimulant, Insect Repellant, Insecticide, Rubefacient

Traditional Use:
Cajeput has been added to household cleansing preparations to help reduce bacteria and viruses on solid and soft surfaces.
Cajeput is traditionally used in air purification treatments to cleanse the air of bacteria and viruses.

Cajuput is used as part of a traditional aromatic treatment for the relief of sinus and chest congestion associated with conditions like bronchitis, colds, allergies, and pneumonia and to help shorten the duration or lessen the severity of common infections.

Part Used:
Leaves, Twigs

Side Effects:
Cajeput is not recommended for use by women who are pregnant or nursing.

Cajeput is not recommended in children's treatments.

Cajeput is not recommended for use by people with kidney problems.

Cajeput may worsen asthma symptoms in some people.

Cajeput may cause skin irritation. You should dilute it before applying Cajeput to the skin and it is not recommended for use in the facial area.

Additional uses and side effects may exist but further research is necessary to determine the exact properties and effects of use.

General:
Cajeput is native to Australia and Asia preferring extremely wet conditions for optimal growth.

Cajeput oil is extracted from the leaves and twigs of the tree and blended with other oils for use as a traditional supplement diluted at 5 drops Cajeput to 1-tablespoon carrier oil.

Camu Camu, Cacari, Camo Camo, Rumberry

Botanical Name:
Myrciaria dubia

Properties:
Antibacterial, Antioxidant, Antiviral, Balancing, Immunostimulant, Neuroprotective

Traditional Uses:

Camu Camu is traditionally used in supplements to protect against and treat common bacterial and viral infections.

Camu Camu contains large amounts of vitamin C and is used as a traditional preparation to help strengthen the immune system.

Parts Used:
Fruit, Leaf

Side Effects:
Camu Camu is not recommended for use by women who are pregnant or nursing.

Additional uses and side effects may exist but further research is necessary to determine the exact properties and effects of use.

General:
Camu Camu is native to the rainforests of South America and has been cultivated indoors in other regions. Camu Camu requires damp, warm surroundings in order to thrive and it can be propagated by seeds or division of the suckers in the spring.

The fruit is used as a food and the fruit and leaves are harvested for use in traditional supplements.

Carline Thistle, Carlina, Dwarf Carline, Ground Thistle, Stemless Carline

Botanical Name:
Carlina acaulis

Properties:
Antibacterial, Antibiotic, Antifungal, Antiseptic, Antispasmodic, Antiviral, Carminative, Diaphoretic, Diuretic, Emetic, Febrifuge, Vermifuge

Traditional Use:
The essential oils of the Carline root have shown some antiviral activity and are used in traditional supplements to treat colds, influenza, and other common infections.

The essential oil of the Carline Thistle root has antibacterial and antiviral properties and has been incorporated into household cleaners.

The essential oil of the Carline Thistle root have been incorporated into steam based air purification recipes to eliminate bacteria and viruses in the home.

Part Used:
Root - Oil

Side Effects:
Carline Thistle is not recommended for use by women who are pregnant or nursing.

Carline Thistle may cause an allergic reaction in some people.

Overuse of Carline Thistle is purgative.

Additional uses and side effects may exist but further research is necessary to determine the exact properties and effects of use.

General:
Carline Thistle is native to Europe and naturalized to North America. Hardy to zone 4, it is not particular regarding soil composition but does prefer full sun and consistent moisture. It is propagated by seed surface sown in the spring.

Carline Thistle flowering heads are eaten as a cooked vegetable and the root and stems are peeled and steamed. The root is harvested in the fall and dried for use in tea traditionally given at a rate of 2 teaspoons root powder to 1 cup of water 3 times daily. The root is also steam distilled to extract the essential oils.

Cat's Claw, Life Giving Vine, Garabato, Healing Vine, Samento, Una de Gato, Vilcacora

Botanical Name:
Uncaria tomentosa

Properties:
Abortifacient, Analgesic, Antibacterial, Antifungal, Anti-inflammatory, Antioxidant, Antiviral, Cancer, Contraceptive, Diuretic, Hypotensive, Immunostimulant, Vasodilator, Vermifuge

Traditional Use:
Cat's Claw s antiviral action make it a traditional supplement treatment for relief from cold sores, herpes, shingles, and other viral related diseases.

Alkaloids in Cat's Claw are used in traditional preparations to stimulate the immune system aiding the white blood cells in fighting off disease.

Part Used:
Inner Bark, Leaf, Root, Stem

Side Effects:
Cat's Claw is not recommended for use by women who are pregnant, nursing or trying to become pregnant because cat's claw has been used as a contraceptive and abortifacient.

Cat's Claw is not recommended for use by people with low blood pressure.

Cat's Claw is not recommended for use by people who have an autoimmune disorder like Multiple Sclerosis or Lupus.

Cat's Claw is not recommended for use by people who have leukemia.

Overuse of Cat's Claw may cause headaches, dizziness, and vomiting.

Additional uses and side effects may exist but further research is necessary to determine the exact properties and effects of use.

General:
Cat's claw is a vine native to Central and South America and prefers to grow on trees in the canopy layer of the rainforest. The inner bark, roots, and stem of Cat's Claw is most commonly used as a tea traditionally taken up to 3 times day but is also available as an extract or capsule supplement. Add 1 tsp of lemon juice to release the tannins in the herb. Do not confusion Cat's Claw Uncaria tomentosa with Cat's Claw Uncaria guianensis.

Chanca Piedra, Amli, Bhonya, Cane Peas, Cane Senna, Creole Senna, Hurricane Weed, Jar Amla, Mapatan, Quebrapedera, Quinine Weed, Rami Buah, Sasha Foster, Shatter Stone, Stone Breaker, Tamalaka

Botanical Name:
Phyllanthus niruri

Properties:
Antibacterial, Anti-inflammatory, Antispasmodic, Antiviral, Diuretic, Emmenagogue, Febrifuge, Hypoglycemic, Immunostimulant

Traditional Use:
Chanca Piedra has traditionally been used in supplements to help shorten the duration and intensity of common viral infections like influenza and hepatitis B and is being researched to determine other potential applications for its antiviral properties.

Part Used:
Flower, Leaf

Side Effects:

Chanca Piedra is not recommended for use by women who are pregnant or nursing.

Chanca Piedra may affect blood sugar.

Additional uses and side effects may exist but further research is necessary to determine the exact properties and effects of use.

General:
Chanca Piedra is a common tropical plant and is considered an invasive species in some regions. Hardy to zone 6, It is not particular regarding soil or sun conditions but does prefer consistent moisture. It can be propagated by seeds soaked and sown in the spring and will self-sow readily if given its own place in the garden.

The supplement benefits of the plant are usually extracted using a water bath method and taken as a tincture. Chanca Piedra has been used for thousands of years as a traditional supplement and is being researched for inclusion in commercial pharmaceuticals.

Cimicifuga, Bugbane

Botanical Name:
Cimicifuga heracleifolia

Properties:
Analgesic, Antibacterial, Antiviral, Sedative

Traditional Use:
Cimicifuga has traditionally been used to promote rest and ease the pain associated with infections like the common cold and influenza while acting to reduce the duration and severity of the related viral infection.

Part Used:
Root

Side Effects:

Cimicifuga is not recommended for use by women who are pregnant or nursing.

Additional uses and side effects may exist but further research is necessary to determine the exact properties and effects of use.

General:
Cimicifuga is native to Asia. Hardy to zone 3, it is not particular regarding soil composition but prefers partial shade and consistent moisture. Cimicifuga can be propagated by seed sown as soon as it is ripe or spring division.

The root is harvested for use fresh or dried and powdered for use in traditional decoctions.

Cinnamon, Cannelle de Ceylan, Cassia Bark

Botanical Name:
Cinnamomum zeylanicum

Properties:
Analgesic, Anti-inflammatory, Antibacterial, Antifungal, Antimicrobial, Antioxidant, Antiperspirant, Antispasmodic, Antiviral, Aphrodisiac, Astringent, Cancer, Deodorant, Digestive, Estrogenic, Hypotensive, Insect Repellant, Stimulant

Traditional Use:
Cinnamon oil is used in cleaning products to reduce fungus and bacteria. A recent study indicates that cinnamon oil has antimicrobial properties that make it effective against certain infections like streptococcus, staphylococcus, & drug resistant infections like MRSA. Cinnamon is traditionally blended with other oils like thyme, lemon, and lemon grass to make an effective disinfectant.

Cinnamon has traditionally been used in supplements to prevent or shorten the severity and number of viral infections like the common cold and influenza.

Part Used:
Bark, Leaf, Oil

Side Effects:
Cinnamon is not recommended for use beyond dietary by women who are pregnant or nursing.

Cinnamon oil may be irritating to the skin and should be handled with care and diluted in any remedy.

Cinnamon may lower blood sugar.

Additional uses and side effects may exist but further research is necessary to determine the exact properties and effects of use.

General:
Cinnamon is a common culinary additive grown in hot, tropical climates and used worldwide. Cinnamon bark is also harvested, dried, and used as a traditional supplement tea.

Clematis, Old Man's Beard, Traveler's Joy, Virgin's Bower

Botanical Name:
Clematis recta, Clematis virginiana

Properties:
Anti-inflammatory, Antimicrobial, Antiviral, Astringent

Traditional Use:
Clematis is traditionally incorporated into topical ointments, washes, and creams for the treatment of herpes and syphilis sores.

Part Used:
Flower, Leaf, Stem

Side Effects:
Clematis is not recommended for use by women who are pregnant or nursing.

Clematis is poison and should not be used internally. Internal use may cause confusion, convulsions, and dizziness.

Overuse of clematis may cause serious skin burns, blisters, or hyper pigmentation.

Additional uses and side effects may exist but further research is necessary to determine the exact properties and effects of use.

General:
Clematis is native to Europe but is cultivated in other regions including the United States. The fresh, flowering plant is harvested for use fresh in external applications. Clematis is not used internally.

Clove, Ding Xiang, Girofle, Kreteks, Lavanga

Botanical Name:
Syzygium aromaticum

Properties:
Anodyne, Antibacterial, Antifungal, Antioxidant, Antiperspirant, Antiseptic, Antispasmodic, Antiviral, Aphrodisiac, Carminative, Digestive, Headache, Hypoglycemic, Insect Repellant, Stimulant, Tonic

Traditional Use:
Clove is almost pure eugenol that is a photochemical that numbs pain while acting to kill bacteria, viruses, and fungus making it a traditional choice for household cleaners and for treatments for bacterial, fungal, and viral infections.

Clove has been used as a traditional supplement to reduce the duration and severity of viral infections such as colds and influenza.

Clove oil is traditionally added to vapor or diffuser preparations to cleanse the air and help ward off common winter infections

Clove oil is added to aromatherapy lamps, room cleaners, and vaporizers as a disinfecting agent.

Part Used:
Flower, Leaf, Stem - Oil

Side Effects:
Clove is not recommended for use beyond dietary by women who are pregnant or nursing.

Clove is not recommended for use beyond dietary by people who are taking blood-thinning medication or who have a bleeding disorder.

Clove oil is highly irritating to the skin and should be handled with caution.

Clove may cause an allergic reaction in some people.

Clove may increase the allergic reactions to other irritants in some people.

Clove may lower blood sugar.

Additional uses and side effects may exist but further research is necessary to determine the exact properties and effects of use.

General:
Clove is the flower from Syzygium aromaticum native to Indonesia but cultivated in many areas of the world. Clove is not particular regarding soil composition but does prefer high moisture and plentiful sun.

Cloves are used as a spice worldwide and have been smoked as a tobacco alternative. Clove is a common ingredient in insect repelling preparations and is especially effective against ants.

The flowers are harvested before blooming and dried or the oils are extracted from the flowers for use in traditional aromatherapy or topical preparations.

Columbine, Culverwort, European Columbine, Granny's Nightcap

Botanical Name:
Aquilegia vulgaris

Properties:
Anodyne, Antibacterial, Antifungal, Antiviral, Astringent, Diuretic, Diaphoretic, Insecticide, Nervine, Sedative

Traditional Use:
Columbine has been used in traditional supplements to treat bacterial, fungal, and viral infections including staphylococcus aureus, micrococcus luteus, bacillus subtilus, and candida albicans, and all strains of influenza.

Part Used:
Leaf, Flower, Stem

Side Effects:
Columbine is not recommended for use by women who are pregnant or nursing.

Overuse of Columbine may be toxic.

Additional uses and side effects may exist but further research is necessary to determine the exact properties and effects of use.

General:
Columbine is native to Asia and Europe and has been naturalized to the United States. Hardy to zone 3, it prefers sandy to loamy soil with full to partial sun and consistent moisture. Columbine is propagated by seeds sown out as soon as they are ripe.

The aerial parts of the plant are harvested while in bloom and dried and powdered for use in a traditional teas or topical preparations.

Corncockle, Cockle, Corn Campion, Corn Cockle, Corn Rose, Crown of the Field

Botanical Name:

Agrostemma githago

Properties:
Antibacterial, Antiviral, Diuretic, Expectorant, Vermifuge

Traditional Uses:
Corncockle is traditionally used in topical ointments to help kill bacteria, viruses, and parasites.

Parts Used:
Root, Seed

Side Effects:
Corncockle is not recommended for use by women who are pregnant or nursing.

The leaves and seeds of the Corncockle are toxic and are not recommended for internal use. The sapopins may be absorbed through the skin and should be used only under the guidance of a qualified herbalist or physician.

Corn Cockle is for external use only. Internal use may cause breathing difficulty, diarrhea, dizziness, paralysis, vomiting, coma, and even death.

Additional uses and side effects may exist but further research is necessary to determine the exact properties and effects of use.

General:
Corncockle is an annual plant native to Asia & Europe but naturalized in other areas where it is considered an invasive weed by some. It is not particular regarding soil composition but prefers full to partial sun and dry to moist conditions. Corncockle can be found growing wild in cornfields or propagated by seeds sown out as soon as they are ripe.

The leaves have been cooked as a vegetable and the root & seed have been harvested for use in traditional supplements.

Cubeb, Cubbebs, Java Pepper, Kabeb Chini, Kankol, Sheetal, Tailed Chubebs, Tailed Pepper

Botanical Name:
Piper cuberba

Properties:
Antiseptic, Antiviral, Astringent, Carminative, Diuretic, Expectorant, Stimulant

Traditional Use:
The astringent & expectorant action of Cubeb has traditionally been used to tone the mucus membranes while expelling excess mucus in congestive disorders like asthma, chronic bronchitis, colds and influenza while the antiviral action works at shortening the duration of related infection.

Cubeb oil has been used to kill common viruses and research indicates that it is effective against influenza.

Part Used:
Unripe Fruit, Oil

Side Effects:
Cubeb is not recommended for use by women who are pregnant or nursing.

Additional uses and side effects may exist but further research is necessary to determine the exact properties and effects of use.

General:
Cubeb is native to Indonesia but is cultivated in other regions where the fruit is harvested just before ripening, dried, and powdered for use in traditional preparations at a rate of ¼ ounce of powder daily or the oils extracted for use in traditional supplement preparations.

Cucumber – Chinese, Chinese Cucumber, Chinese Snake Gourd, Gua Lua, Tian Hua Fen

Botanical Name:
Trichosanthes japonica

Properties:
Abortifacient, Antibacterial, Anti-inflammatory, Antiviral, Hypoglycemic

Traditional Uses:
A compound in Chinese Cucumber has been used in traditional supplements to treat viruses including HIV and it is believed to attack the virus at a different point than AZT.

Parts Used:
Fruit, Root, Seed

Side Effects:
Chinese Cucumber should not be used without the advice of a qualified herbalist or physician.

Chinese Cucumber is not recommended for use by women who are pregnant or nursing.

The root and seed of the Chinese Cucumber have been used as an abortifacient.

Chinese Cucumber is not recommended for use by people with diabetes.

Additional uses and side effects may exist but further research is necessary to determine the exact properties and effects of use.

General:
Chinese Cucumber is native to Asia and has been used in traditional Chinese supplements for thousands of years. The root and seed have been harvested for use in topical and supplement treatments and an extract has been isolated that is being researched for potential cancer and HIV related treatments.

Devil's Club, Cukilanarpak, Devil's Root, Fatsia

Botanical Name:
Echinopanax horridum

Properties:
Antibacterial, Antifungal, Antiviral, Expectorant, Stimulant

Traditional Uses:
Devil's Club has been used as a traditional supplement to stimulate the respiratory tract, soften and expel mucus in congestive conditions like asthma, bronchitis, colds, influenza, and pneumonia while acting to kill the underlying infection.

Devil's Club has antiviral properties that have made it a traditional component in supplements to shorten the duration and severity of common infections like the common cold and influenza.

Devil's Club is traditionally included in liquid preparations to kill bacteria, fungus, and viruses on the skin and in surface cleaners.

Parts Used:
Inner Root Bark

Side Effects:
Devil's Club is not recommended for use by women who are pregnant or nursing.

Devil's Club may affect blood sugar.

Additional uses and side effects may exist but further research is necessary to determine the exact properties and effects of use.

General:
The root of the Devil's Claw is harvested and peeled so that the inner root can be dried, powdered, and incorporated into topical preparations or for supplement uses. The essential oils are extracted for use in liquid preparations.

Dragon's Blood

Botanical Name:
Croton lechleri

Properties:
Antiviral, Astringent, Styptic

Traditional Use:
Dragon's Blood has been used as part of a traditional treatment to prevent or shorten the severity and duration of common viral infections especially respiratory infections like influenza.

Part Used:
Resin

Side Effects:
Dragon's Blood is not recommended for use by women who are pregnant or nursing.

Additional uses and side effects may exist but further research is necessary to determine the exact properties and effects of use.

General:
Dragon's Blood is the resin of the Dragon Tree found in many tropical and sub-tropical regions around the world.

The resin is harvested from the ripe fruit for use as a color varnish, dye product, and both commercial pharmaceuticals and traditional supplements.

The active compound is extracted in an alcohol bath.

Do not confuse Dragon's Blood Croton lechleri with Dragon's Blood Daemonorops draco.

Dragons Blood, Sangre

Botanical Name:

Daemonorops draco

Properties:
Antioxidant, Antiviral, Astringent, Colorant, Hallucinogenic

Traditional Use:
Dragon's Blood has been used as part of a traditional treatment to prevent or shorten the severity and duration of common viral infections especially respiratory infections like influenza.

Part Used:
Bark, Resin

Side Effects:
Dragon's Blood is not recommended for use by women who are pregnant or nursing.

Dragon's Blood is not recommended for internal use or as smoked incense as it is believed to have hallucinogenic properties.

Additional uses and side effects may exist but further research is necessary to determine the exact properties and effects of use.

General:
Dragon's Blood is the resin of the Dragon Tree found in many tropical and sub-tropical regions around the world. The Dragon Tree is a type of palm hardy to zone 10b. It is not particular regarding sun conditions but does prefer a moist environment and rich soil.

The stems are used in woodcraft making items like canes and furniture. The resin and red leaves have been smoked or eaten in religious ceremonies. The resin is harvested from the ripe fruit for use as a color varnish, dye product, and both commercial pharmaceuticals and traditional supplements where the active compounds are extracted in an alcohol bath. Do not confuse Dragon's Blood Daemonorops draco with Dragon's Blood Croton lechleri.

Echinacea, Black Samson, Purple Coneflower

Botanical Name:
Echinacea angustifolia, Echinacea purpurea

Properties:
Adaptogen, Antibacterial, Anti-inflammatory, Antiseptic, Antibacterial, Antiviral, Depurative, Digestive, Immunostimulant

Traditional Use:
All types of Echinacea contain compounds that support disease resistance and are traditionally used to help to shorten the length of common infections when taken as soon as symptoms appears.

Extracts of Echinacea root have shown immunostimulatory effects in clinical trails and Echinacea has been used as a traditional supplement to inhibit viruses and increase antibacterial and microphage activity.

Echinacea is traditionally used to reduce the number, severity, and duration of herpes virus outbreaks including cold sores.

Echinacea extract is being studied for the prevention of genital herpes outbreaks.

Echinacea has traditionally been used to help to alleviate inflammation of the mucus membranes of the digestive and respiratory system and to alleviate the pain of a sore throat or tonsils while combating infection.

Part Used:
Flower, Leaf, Root, Stem

Side Effects:
Echinacea is not recommended for use by women who are pregnant or nursing.

Echinacea may cause an allergic reaction, skin rash, or gastrointestinal upset in some people.

Echinacea is not recommended for use by people who have an autoimmune disease like Multiple Sclerosis or Lupus.

Overuse of Echinacea may cause fever, nausea, and vomiting.

Extended use of Echinacea may cause immunosuppression.

Additional uses and side effects may exist but further research is necessary to determine the exact properties and effects of use.

General:
There are nine known species of Echinacea native to the United States & Canada. The most potent species are Echinacea angustifolia (white flower) and Echinacea purpurea (purple flower). Hardy to zone 3, Echinacea is drought resistant once established but requires full sun for optimal growth. It can be propagated by seed sown out in the spring, spring division, or root cuttings in the late fall.

The entire plant including flower, leaf, root, and stem are used to make teas, juice, extracts or in preparations for external use. The root contains the highest concentration of beneficial compounds. Therapeutic levels of Echinacea are delivered in tincture form at a rate of 50 drops up to 5 times daily.

Edelweiss, Lion's Paw, Queen's Flower

Botanical Name:
Leontopodium alpinum

Properties:
Antibacterial, Anti-inflammatory, Antiviral, Antimicrobial, Antioxidant

Traditional Use:
Edelweiss has traditionally been used as part of natural cleaning products to kill bacteria and viruses in the air and on hard surfaces.

Edelweiss has been used as a traditional supplement to help shorten the length of common respiratory infections like colds and influenza.

Side Effects:

Edelweiss is not recommended for use by women who are pregnant or nursing.

Additional uses and side effects may exist but further research is necessary to determine the exact properties and effects of use.

General:
Edelweiss can be found growing in higher altitudes and is cultivated as an ornamental or for disinfectant and supplement uses.

Elder, Baccae, Black Elder, Elderberry, Ellanwood, Ellhorn, European Alder, Holunderbeeren, Sambucus, Sauco, Sureau

Botanical Name:
Sambucus

Properties:
Anti-inflammatory, Antimicrobial, Antiviral, Astringent, Cancer, Colorant, Depurative, Diuretic, Emollient, Expectorant, Laxative, Immunostimulant

Traditional Use:
Elder flowers are used as a traditional infusion to reduce bronchial and upper respiratory constriction and help to expel excess mucus in congestive disorders like asthma, bronchitis, colds, influenza, and pneumonia while acting to fight any underlying infection.

Elder berries have traditionally been used to help reduce the length and severity of common infections like colds & influenza.

Aged Elder bark contains active compounds that inhibit the enzymes that influenza viruses use to penetrate our cell membranes making the flower and berry combination a traditional treatment for the prevention of common influenza infections and the juice has been used to reduce the length of the flu virus.

Part Used:
Bark, Flower

Side Effects:
Elder is not recommended for use by women who are pregnant or nursing.

Elder is not recommended for use by people who have an autoimmune disease like Multiple Sclerosis or Lupus.

Unripe or uncooked elder berries are toxic and may cause nausea, vomiting, and diarrhea.

Fresh Elder Bark is toxic. Only aged bark is used for traditional supplements.

Elder flowers have diuretic effects and should not be used by those taking drugs to increase urination.

Additional uses and side effects may exist but further research is necessary to determine the exact properties and effects of use.

General:
Elder is native to Europe and North America but has been cultivated in other regions. Hardy to zone 6, it is not particular regarding soil composition but does prefer full to partial shade and consistent moisture. Elder can be propagated by seed sown out in the spring or by cuttings taken in mid-summer. Suckers can be separated during the dormant season.

The dried flowers and cooked berries of the Elder are traditionally used in teas, extracts, and capsule form with a traditional infusion preparation being 2 teaspoon of dried flower to 1-cup boiling water 8 times daily.

Elecampane, Alant, Aster, Elfdock, Elfwort, Horse Elder, Horseheal, Indian Elecampane, Scabwort, Velvet Dock, Wild Sunflower, Yellow Starwort

Botanical Name: Inula helenium

Properties: Analgesic, Antibacterial, Antifungal, Anti-inflammatory, Antimicrobial, Antiseptic, Astringent, Cholagogue, Colorant, Demulcent, Detoxification, Diaphoretic, Diuretic, Expectorant, Vermifuge

Traditional Use: The ooze of the Elecampane root has traditionally been used in steam treatments to cleanse the air of common bacteria, fungus, and viruses.

Elecampane is traditionally used in surface, air, and wound cleaning products to kill bacteria, fungus, and viruses.

Part Used: Flower, Rhizome, Root

Side Effects: Elecampane is not recommended for use by women who are pregnant or nursing.

Elecampane may cause allergies to people sensitive to plants in the sunflower family.

Elecampane may irritate the mucus membranes.

Elecampane may affect blood sugar.

Additional uses and side effects may exist but further research is necessary to determine the exact properties and effects of use.

General: Elecampane is a perennial native to Europe and naturalized in many other areas of the world. It is not particular regarding soil composition but does prefer full or partial sun and consistent moisture. Elecampane grows easily from root cuttings or seed.

Elephant Tree

Botanical Name:
Bursera microphylla

Properties:
Antibacterial, Antiviral, Astringent, Expectorant, Immunostimulant

Traditional Use:
Elephant Tree bark, leaf, and resin have traditionally been used as a stimulating expectorant for congestive conditions like asthma, bronchitis,

cough, and influenza while acting to reduce the length and severity of common infections.

Elephant Tree bark, leaves, and resin have traditionally been used in alcohol tinctures to alleviate pain and inflammation while reducing infection and speeding healing in cold sores, mouth sores, and tooth abscesses.

Elephant Tree leaves have been used as a traditional supplement tea to help build the immune system and ward off common infections.

Part Used:
Bark, Leaf, Resin

Side Effects:
Elephant Tree is not recommended for use by women who are pregnant or nursing.

Additional uses and side effects may exist but further research is necessary to determine the exact properties and effects of use.

General:
Elephant Tree is a small shrub native to Central America and the southern United States. The resin is harvested for use in varnish products and the bark, leaf and resin are harvested, dried, and powdered for use as a traditional supplement.

Ephedra – Joint Fir, Ephedra, Joint Fir Ephedra, Sea Grape

Botanical Name:
Ephedra distachya

Properties:
Antispasmodic, Antitussive, Antiviral, Diaphoretic, Diuretic, Febrifuge, Hypertensive, Nervine, Tonic, Vasoconstrictor

Traditional Use:

Joint Fir Ephedra has been used as a traditional treatment to prevent or shorten the duration and severity of viral infections like influenza and has shown the ability in laboratory studies to combat influenza viruses.

Part Used:
Leaf, Stem

Side Effects:
The FDA banned the U.S. sale of dietary supplements containing Ephedra. Ephedra has been banned for use in dietary substances in the United States. Ephedra affects the brains and central nervous system in the same way as amphetamines but not as powerfully. Since Ephedra works as a stimulant, it affects the heart and blood pressure and has lost much of its appeal as a supplement. The FDA found that these supplements had a high risk of injury or illness and a risk of death. The ban does not apply to traditional Chinese herbal remedies or to products like herbal teas that are regulated as conventional foods.

Joint Fir Ephedra should only be used under the guidance of a qualified herbalist or physician.

Joint Fir Ephedra is not recommended for use by women who are pregnant or nursing.

Joint Fir Ephedra affects the brain and central nervous system in the same way as amphetamines but not as powerfully.

Joint Fir Ephedra is not recommended for use by people who have high blood pressure, hyperthyroidism, or glaucoma or who are taking MOAI inhibitors.

Additional uses and side effects may exist but further research is necessary to determine the exact properties and effects of use.

General:
Joint Fir Ephedra is an evergreen shrub native to semi-desert and desert regions of Asia and Europe. Hardy to zone 6, it prefers sandy to loamy soil and requires full sun and consistent moisture. Joint Fir can be propagated by seeds sown as soon as they are ripe, division in the spring, or layering.

Joint Fir fruits are eaten raw and the leaf and stem are harvested for use fresh or in traditional teas, extracts, or tinctures.

Eucalyptus, Blue Gum Blue Mallee, Gully Gum, Gum Tree, Red Gum, Stringy Bark Tree, Sagandhapara

Botanical Name: Eucalyptus globulus

Properties: Analgesic, Antibacterial, Antifungal, Anti-inflammatory, Antiperspirant, Antiseptic, Antispasmodic, Antiviral, Astringent, Cancer, Colorant, Depurative, Diuretic, Expectorant, Febrifuge, Hypoglycemic, Insect Repellant, Rubefacient, Vermifuge

Traditional Use: Eucalyptus is a traditional decongestant that opens the lungs, clears clogged nasal passages, and loosens phlegm making it a component in traditional allergy, asthma, bronchitis, cold, and influenza treatments while acting to shorten the duration and severity of related infection. It is used as a traditional supplement tincture or tea or as part of a vapor inhalant therapy.

Eucalyptus oils is a powerful antiseptic have been used in natural cleaning products as an agent to kill airborne or surface bacteria, viruses, and fungus.

Part Used: Leaf, Oil

Side Effects: Eucalyptus is not recommended for use by women who are pregnant or nursing.

Eucalyptus is not recommended for use in children's treatments.

Eucalyptus is not recommended for use by people with a history of seizure disorders.

Eucalyptus may lower blood sugar.

Undiluted Eucalyptus oil is toxic both internally and externally. Always dilute Eucalyptus Oil before use. The leaf is generally considered safe in teas.

Overuse of Eucalyptus oil may cause difficulty breathing, dizziness, gastrointestinal irritation, hallucinations, nausea, vomiting, paralysis, convulsions, and even death.

Additional uses and side effects may exist but further research is necessary to determine the exact properties and effects of use.

General: Eucalyptus is native to Australia but is cultivated in many other parts of the world. Hardy to zone 9, it is not particular regarding soil composition but does prefer full sun and moist to wet conditions. Eucalyptus can be propagated by seeds sown after all danger of frost has passed. If sown indoors, seedlings should be transplanted to their permanent location as soon as the second set of leaves appear.

Eucalyptus leaf oil is used in insect repelling preparations. According to the CDC, Lemon Eucalyptus has proven to be as effective as DEET at repelling insects like mosquitoes. The oils are also used as a cleanser effective against grease, bacteria, and a variety of fungal growths. The wood is valued for indoor and outdoor woodcraft or pulped for making paper. The young leaves yield a self-mordanting yellow to tan colorant, the young shoots yield tones of grey to green and the young bark yields a darker green. Eucalyptus is one of the most commonly used treatments for cough, congestion, and household disinfecting cleaners. The oil is extracted from fresh or partially dried leaves for use in aromatherapy and traditional supplements.

Fo-Ti, Chinese Cornbind, Chinese Knotweed, Climbing Knotweed, Flowery Knotweed, He-Shou-Wu, Tuber Fleeceflower

Botanical Name: Polygonum multiflorum

Properties: Adaptogen, Analgesic, Antibacterial, Antioxidant, Antispasmodic, Astringent, Cancer, Cardiotonic, Detoxification, Hypoglycemic, Hypotensive, Laxative, Phytoestrogen, Sedative, Skin Care, Tonic

Traditional Use: Fo Ti has traditionally been used to stimulate the immune system and to ward off viruses or bacterial infections.

Part Used: Root, Stem

Side Effects: Fo Ti is not recommended for use by women who are pregnant or nursing.

Fo Ti is not recommended for use in children's treatments.

Fo-Ti may increase blood sugar.

Fo Ti is not recommended for use by people liver or kidney disease without the guidance of a qualified herbalist or physician.

Overdose or overuse of Fo Ti may cause numbness, tingling in the extremities, abdominal pain, diarrhea, and nausea.

Additional uses and side effects may exist but further research is necessary to determine the exact properties and effects of use.

General: Fo-Ti is native to China and Japan and can be found growing along forest edges and open fields. Hardy to zone 7, it is not particular regarding soil composition but does prefer full to partial sun and consistent moisture. Fo-Ti can be propagated by seed sown out in the spring or through division of the clumps.

Fo-Ti leaves and seeds are eaten raw or cooked and the root is soaked to remove the bitterness and then eaten as a cooked vegetable. Fo-Ti is a very popular traditional supplement in China where the roots are harvested in the fall, dried, and powdered or steam processed for use as a traditional supplement with the most mature roots holding the most supplement value. The stems are harvested in the fall and used fresh or dried and powdered for use in traditional infusions. Extracts of the entire plant have been used in traditional cancer treatment plans.

Fennel, Biri Sanuf, Bitter Fennel, Carosella, Hinojo, Sweet Fennel, Wild Fennel, Xiao Hui Xiang

Botanical Name: Foeniculum vulgare

Properties: Adaptogenic, Analgesic, Anodyne, Antidepressant, Antifungal, Antiinflammatory, Antimicrobial, Antiseptic, Antispasmodic, Antiviral, Appetite Depressant, Carminative, Colorant, Depurative, Detoxification, Diaphoretic, Diuretic, Emmenagogue, Estrogenic, Expectorant, Galactagogue, Hallucinogenic, Insect Repellant, Laxative, Vulnerary

Traditional Use: Fennel tea or syrup contains more creosol and alpha-pinene than anise making it a traditional supplement for helping the body expel excess mucus and in calming dry coughs in conditions like asthma, bronchitis, colds, influenza and sinusitis while acting to treat the underlying infection.

Fennel has been included in traditional sprays & gargles to alleviate throat & mouth inflammation and infection.

Fennel oil has antiviral properties and is used in air purifiers to clear the air of viral infections.

Part Used: Leaf, Oil, Root, Seed, Whole

Side Effects: Fennel is not recommended for use by women who are pregnant or nursing.

Fennel is a uterine stimulant.

Fennel may cause photosensitivity, indigestion, pulmonary edema, and vomiting.

Fennel is not recommended for use by women who have an estrogen sensitive disorder like endometriosis, fibroids or certain types of cancer.

Fennel can affect blood sugar.

Fennel oil may affect liver function.

Additional uses and side effects may exist but further research is necessary to determine the exact properties and effects of use.

General:
Fennel is an annual plant native to the Mediterranean but is cultivated worldwide as it is easily grown from seed in rich soil with plenty of sun and moderate moisture. It grows to a height of 3-6 feet and has yellow flowers that bloom in the summer months. Fennel should be grown away from other plants since it may inhibit their growth.

Fennel leaves, stalks, and flower heads are eaten as a raw or cooked vegetable and the seeds are used as an anise-like flavoring. Dried fennel leaves have been used as part of insect repellant powders especially to protect pets against fleas.

The leaf and root are harvested for use fresh or dried and powdered for use in traditional supplements. The oils are extracted from the crushed seed for use in topical and aromatherapy treatments.

Forsythia, Forsitia, Golden Bell, Lian Qiao, Lien Chiao, Rengyo, Yellow Bell, Weeping Golden Bell

Botanical Name:
Forsythia suspensa

Properties:
Antibacterial, Anti-inflammatory, Antitussive, Antiviral, Antiseptic, Astringent, Cancer, Diuretic, Emmenagogue, Febrifuge, Natural Skin Care, Vermifuge

Traditional Use:
Forsythia is traditionally used to reduce inflammation in the small bronchial passages and has been used as a traditional treatment for asthma, bronchitis, colds, and influenza while acting to reduce the duration and severity of the underlying infection.

Forsythia fruit tea is traditionally used as a tea to ward off or shorten the duration and severity of viral infections particularly colds and influenza.

Part Used:
Flower, Leaf, Twig

Side Effects:
Forsythia is not recommended for use by women who are pregnant or nursing.

Additional uses and side effects may exist but further research is necessary to determine the exact properties and effects of use.

General: Forsythia is native to Asia but is now found in many regions of the world. Hardy to zone 5, it is not particular regarding soil composition or sun conditions but does prefer consistent moisture. Forsythia can be propagated by seeds sown in the spring, cutting, air layering, or division.

Forsythia has been used as a traditional supplement for thousands of years and the twigs, fruit, and leaves have been harvested, dried, and powdered for use internally and externally.

Garden Cress, Cress, Pepper Grass

Botanical Name:
Lepidium sativum

Properties:
Abortifacient, Antibacterial, Antiviral, Diuretic, Expectorant, Galactogogue, Immunostimulant

Traditional Use:
Garden Cress has traditionally been used to calm coughs and congestion associated with asthma, bronchitis, colds, and influenza and as a component in traditional supplements to shorten the length of common bacterial and viral infections.

Garden Cress is rich in Vitamin C and is traditionally used in conditions arising from a Vitamin C deficiency and has shown high levels of antibacterial and antiviral effects in laboratory testing leading to its inclusion in immunity related therapy.

Part Used:
Flower, Leaf, Stem

Side Effects:
Garden Cress was traditionally used as an abortifacient and should never be used by a pregnant or nursing woman.

The oil of the plant may cause skin irritation, blisters, and even necrosis.

Additional uses and side effects may exist but further research is necessary to determine the exact properties and effects of use.

General:
Garden Cress is an annual grown in many parts of the world as a food. Hardy to zone 7, it is not particular regarding soil composition but does prefer full to partial sun and consistent moisture. Garden Cress can be propagated by seed sown in the spring.

Garden Cress seeds yield edible oil used in candle making and lighting. The leaf is eaten as a raw or cooked vegetable, the root is used as a condiment, and the seeds are used as a seasoning. The flower, leaf, and stem are harvested during the flowering season for use fresh or as a traditional tea supplement.

Garlic, Allium, Lasuna, Poor Man's Treacle, Rason, Rust Treacle, Stinking Rose

Botanical Name: Allium sativum

Properties: Antibacterial, Antifungal, Antimicrobial, Antioxidant, Antiseptic, Antispasmodic, Astringent, Chalagogue, Cholesterol, Depurative, Diaphoretic, Diuretic, Emmenagogue, Expectorant, Febrifuge, Hypotensive, Immunostimulant, Stimulant, Insect Repellant, Rubefacient, Vermifuge

Traditional Use: Garlic has been used as a traditional supplement to reduce reactivity, minimize coughing and expel excess mucus in congestive conditions like allergies, asthma, colds, bronchitis and influenza while acting to minimize the severity and duration of any underlying infection.

The juices of Garlic have been used as a disinfecting agent in household cleansing products.

Garlic contains a broad spectrum antimicrobial and has traditionally been used in supplements to shorten the length of infections.

Garlic has been used in traditional dietary plans to boost the body's immune response helping to ward off common infections.

Part Used: Bulb, Whole

Side Effects: Garlic is not recommended for use beyond dietary for women who are pregnant or nursing.

Garlic is not recommended for use beyond dietary in children's treatments.

Overuse of Garlic may cause heartburn in some people.

Overuse of Garlic may burn the skin in some people.

Garlic may cause bad breath, body odor, upset stomach, and rarely allergic reactions.

Garlic may reduce blood clotting ability. Do not use garlic supplements if you are planning to have surgery, dental work, or have a bleeding disorder.

Additional uses and side effects may exist but further research is necessary to determine the exact properties and effects of use.

General: Garlic is the edible bulb from a plant in the lily family and has been used as a spice and supplement for thousands of years. Garlic bulbs are traditionally given in high quantities to obtain the supplement value. Two cloves daily is a baseline for supplement use. Garlic can be consumed raw, juiced, or dried into a powder supplement.

The juices of the Garlic have been used as an insect repellant primarily against insects like moths. The bulbs, leaves, and flowers are eaten as a raw or cooked vegetable and the aroma increases as the plant ripens.

Wild Garlic is similar in composition and uses to cultivated Garlic but has a milder aroma and weaker action making it more common for use in traditional treatments given over a longer period. Other types of Garlic including Allium canadense – Canadian Garlic and Allium vineale – Crow Garlic have similar properties with milder aroma and weaker action.

Goldenseal, Eye Balm, Eye Root, Goldenroot, Ground Raspberry, Indian Dye, Indian Plant, Indian Turmeric, Jaundice Root, Orange Root, Turmeric Root, Wild Curcuma, Yellow Indian Pain, Yellow Puccoon, Yellow Root

Botanical Name:
Hydrastis canadensis

Properties:
Antibacterial, Antifungal, Anti-inflammatory, Antiseptic, Antispasmodic, Antiviral, Astringent, Cholagogue, Colorant, Detoxifier, Diuretic, Emmenagogue, Expectorant, Hypoglycemic, Hypotensive, Laxative, Immunostimulant

Traditional Use:
Goldenseal is used in traditional supplements to alleviate the constriction and excess mucus associated with the respiratory conditions allergies, asthma, bronchitis, colds, influenza, and rhinitis while acting to reduce the severity and duration of any underlying infection.

Goldenseal contains berberine that is traditionally used to prevent viruses from invading our cells and causing infections making it a traditional preventative for upper respiratory infections like colds and influenza.

Goldenseal contains active compounds that are used to in traditional preparations to stimulate white blood cells to seek out active infections including bacteria, fungi, viruses, and tumor cells.

Part Used:
Leaf, Root, Underground Stem

Side Effects:
Goldenseal is not recommended for use by women who are pregnant or nursing.

Goldenseal is not recommended for use in children's treatments.

Goldenseal is not intended for long-term use.

Goldenseal contains alkaloids that are toxic in large doses.

Overdose of goldenseal can cause vomiting, diarrhea, or stomach upset in some people.

Goldenseal may lower blood sugar levels, raise blood pressure, or cause gastrointestinal upset.

Goldenseal may change the way your body reacts to other prescription drugs.

Additional uses and side effects may exist but further research is necessary to determine the exact properties and effects of use.

General:
Goldenseal is a perennial native to Eastern North America. Hardy to zone 3, it can be found growing wild in part of the US or cultivated in many supplement gardens. It is not particular regarding soil composition but does prefer full to partial shade and consistent moisture. It can be propagated by seed planted out as soon as they are ripe or by divisions of larger clumps in the fall.

The roots and stalk of the goldenseal yield a yellow colorant used as a textile dye product. The juices pounded out of the roots are used as an insect repellant. The underground stem and root of the Goldenseal plant are harvested in the fall for use fresh or dried, and powdered for use in supplement teas or made into an extract.

Grapefruit, Agume, Shaddock

Botanical Name:
Citrus paradisi

Properties:
Antidepressant, Antifungal, Antioxidant, Antiseptic, Antispasmodic, Antiviral, Diuretic, Stimulant, Tonic

Traditional Use:
Grapefruit seed and inner rind extract is a natural disinfectant included in household cleaners and internal disinfectant remedies at a rate of 3-5 drops per pint of water.

Part Used:
Fruit, Rind, Seed

Side Effects:
Grapefruit is not recommended for use beyond dietary in women who are pregnant or nursing.

Grapefruit may change the way that the body uses estrogen and is not recommended for use by menopausal women or by those who have an estrogen related condition like fibroids, endometriosis, or certain types of cancer.

Grapefruit oil may cause photosensitivity.

Grapefruit may interfere with the function of some over the counter, prescription, and herbal treatments and should not be used without the advice of a qualified herbalist or physician.

Additional uses and side effects may exist but further research is necessary to determine the exact properties and effects of use.

General:
Grapefruit is the fruit of a subtropical citrus tree known as a food throughout the world.

Graviola, Brazilian Cherimoya, Brazilian Paw Paw, Guanabana, Guanavana, Nangka Blanda, Soursop

Botanical Name:
Corossol epineux

Properties:
Antibacterial, Antiparasitic, Antiviral, Cancer, Purgative

Traditional Uses:
Graviola infusions are traditionally used to treat internal and external bacterial and viral infections.

Parts Used:
Leaf, Fruit, Seed

Side Effects:
Graviola is not recommended for use by women who are pregnant or nursing.

Graviola may be cause nerve damage or death.

Graviola may worsen the symptoms of Parkinson's Disease or cause symptoms similar to Parkinson's Disease.

Additional uses and side effects may exist but further research is necessary to determine the exact properties and effects of use.

General:
Graviola is a small evergreen tree native to Brazil where it is harvested and used a seasoning or in beverages. The fruits, leaves, and seeds are also harvested, dried, and powdered for use in traditional supplements.

Guan Jung, Crown Wood Fern

Botanical Name:

Dryopteris crassirhizoma

Properties:
Abortifacient, Analgesic, Antibacterial, Anti-inflammatory, Antioxidant, Antiviral, Astringent, Cancer, Febrifuge, Haemostatic, Vermifuge

Traditional Use:
Guan Jung has been given as a traditional supplement to prevent or shorten the duration and severity of common viral infections like influenza.

Part Used:
Leaf, Root

Side Effects:
Guan Jung is not recommended for use by women who are pregnant or nursing.

Guan Jung has a known abortifacient effect.

Guan Jung should only be used under the care of a qualified herbalist or physician.

Guan Jung roots may be toxic.

Additional uses and side effects may exist but further research is necessary to determine the exact properties and effects of use.

General:
Guan Jung is a fern native to Japan and cultivated as an ornamental in other regions. Hardy to zone 6, it is not particular regarding soil composition but does prefer partial shade and consistent moisture. Guan Jung can be propagated by spores sown in moist conditions or division.

Guan Jung root is harvested in the fall, dried, and powdered for use in traditional supplements. The leaf is harvested during the warm season and made into an alcohol tincture, extract, or dried & powdered for use as a traditional supplement infusion.

Guduchi, Ambervel, Amrita, Gilo, Glunchanb, Gurcha, Indian Tinospora, Jetwatika, Teluga, Tinospora
Botanical Name: Tinsospora cardiofolia

Properties: Adaptogenic, Antibacterial, Antimicrobial, Antiseptic, Astringent, Detoxificant, Hyperglycemic, Immunostimulant, Stimulant, Tonic

Traditional Use: Guduchi has traditionally been given as a treatment component to stimulate the production of white blood cells helping to increase immunity and ward off common infections.

Part Used: Leaf, Root, Stem

Side Effects: Guduchi is not recommended for use by women who are pregnant or nursing.

Guduchi may lower blood sugar.

Additional uses and side effects may exist but further research is necessary to determine the exact properties and effects of use.

General: Guduchi is a semi-parasitic vine native to India and found growing other subtropical regions. It is not particular regarding soil composition but does prefer full to partial sun and dry soil.

The entire plant is harvested, dried, and powdered for use in traditional infusions or the compounds extracted through as a strong decoction.

Gurmar, Gemnema, Gurmarbooti, Miracle Plant, Shardunika, Vishani

Botanical Name:
Gymnema sylvestre

Properties:
Antibacterial, Antiviral, Astringent, Cholesterol, Diuretic, Hypoglycemic

Traditional Use:

Gurmar has shown an ability to kill bacteria and viruses and is often included in household cleaning preparations.

Part Used:
Leaf, Root

Side Effects:
Gurmar is not recommended for use by women who are pregnant or nursing.

Gurmar affects blood sugar.

Additional uses and side effects may exist but further research is necessary to determine the exact properties and effects of use.

General:
Gumar is native to Asia, Africa, and India where the leaves are harvested for use in traditional treatments at a rate of 7-10 grams of powdered leaf per dose.

Hemp Agrimony

Botanical Name:
Eupatorium cannabinum

Properties:
Antiviral, Cancer, Cholagogue, Detoxification, Diaphoretic, Diuretic, Emetic, Expectorant, Febrifuge, Immunostimulant, Laxative, Tonic

Traditional Use:
Hemp Agrimony has been used as a traditional supplement to stimulate the immune system and ward off or treat viral infections shortening the duration and severity of common infections like influenza but it should not be used without the guidance of a qualified herbalist or physician.

Part Used:
Flower, Leaf

Side Effects:
Hemp Agrimony is not recommended for use by women who are pregnant or nursing.

Hemp Agrimony contains compounds that make it unsuitable for use without the guidance of a qualified herbalist or physician.

Overuse of Hemp Agrimony may cause diarrhea, vomiting, or liver damage.

Additional uses and side effects may exist but further research is necessary to determine the exact properties and effects of use.

General:
Hemp Agrimony is a perennial native to Asia but cultivated as an ornamental plant in other regions. Hardy to zone 5, it is not particular regarding soil composition but does prefer full or partial sunlight and consistent moisture. It is easily propagated by seed or by spring division of the clumps.

The leaves are included in insect repellant preparations especially in pet care products. The flower & leaf are harvested, dried, and powdered for use in traditional supplements.

Herb Robert, Crow's Foot, Dove's Foot, Dragon's Blood, Mountain Geranium, Red Robin, Robert Geranium, Stinky Bob, Storksbill, Wild Crane's Bill

Botanical Name:
Geranium robertianum

Properties:
Antibacterial, Antimicrobial, Antiviral, Astringent, Colorant, Diuretic, Hypoglycemic, Vulnerary

Traditional Use:
An extraction of Herb Robert mixed at a rate of 20/80 with ethyl alcohol has traditionally been used to treat infections and has shown an ability to inhibit

or kill common bacteria and viruses including adeno, e. coli, and staphylococcus.

Part Used:
Flower, Leaf, Root, Stem

Side Effects:
Herb Robert is not recommended for use by women who are pregnant or nursing.

Herb Robert may affect blood sugar.

Additional uses and side effects may exist but further research is necessary to determine the exact properties and effects of use.

General:
Herb Robert is native to Africa, Asia, and Europe and naturalized to North and South America. Hardy to zone 6, it is not particular regarding soil composition but does prefer full to partial sun and dry to moist soil. Herb Robert is propagated by seed sown in the spring and will self-sow readily if given its own place in the garden.

Herb Robert yields a brown colorant that has been used as a hair, skin, or textile dye. The colorant extracted as a dye product is used as a sunless tanning lotion that has a secondary benefit of repelling mosquitoes and other biting insects. Herb Robert is harvested during the flowering season and used fresh in traditional supplements or the oils are extracted for later use.

Hibiscus, Gongura, Guinea Sorrel, Jamaica Sorrel, Karkade, Red Sorrel, Red Tea, Roselle, Sour Tea, Sudanease Tea
Botanical Name: Hibiscus sabdariffa

Properties: Antibacterial, Antispasmodic, Antiviral, Astringent, Colorant, Digestive, Diuretic, Emollient, Febrifuge, Hypotensive, Laxative, Sedative, Uterine Relaxant, Vermifuge

Traditional Use: Hibiscus leaves have traditionally been used in topical poultices to alleviate infection in skin sores, ulcers, and abscessed wounds.

The antispasmodic, antiviral, and emollient properties of the Hibiscus flower & leaves have made them a traditional treatment to reduce congestion and treat underlying infections in conditions like asthma, bronchitis, colds, congestion, and influenza.

Part Used: Flower, Leaf, Oil

Side Effects: Hibiscus flower is not recommended for use by women who are pregnant or nursing.

Hibiscus has been used as a uterine relaxant in some cultures.

Hibiscus may lower blood pressure.

Additional uses and side effects may exist but further research is necessary to determine the exact properties and effects of use.

General: Hibiscus is an annual cultivated in many warmer regions as an ornamental and as a container plant in other places. Hardy to zone 10, it is not particular regarding soil composition but does prefer full sun and consistent moisture. Hibiscus is propagated by bulbs planted out in the spring or by division and separation of the bulbs prior to winter storage.

Hibiscus stems are used to make a hemp like fiber. Yellow Hibiscus flowers yield a yellow toned dye.   Red or purple Hibiscus flowers yield a dusky red toned colorant.

Hibiscus flowers are harvested for use in jams, drinks, and foods. The leaves and flowers are harvested and the oils extracted through steam distillation or dried and powdered for use in a traditional supplement tea.

Holy Basil, Ajaka, Baranda, Brinda, Indian Basil, Kemangen, Sacred Basil, Tulsi

Botanical Name: Ocimum sanctum

Properties: Adaptogen, Antibacterial, Antifungal, Anti-inflammatory, Antioxidant, Antitussive, Cancer, Carminative, Cox-2 Inhibitor, Demulcent, Diuretic, Expectorant, Febrifuge, Hypoglycemic, Immunostimulant, Insect Repellant, Laxative

Traditional Use: Holy Basil has traditionally been used to stimulate the immune system helping to ward off common infections.

Part Used: Leaf, Seed, Stem

Side Effects: Holy Basil is not recommended for use by women who are pregnant or nursing.

Holy Basil may slow blood clotting.

Additional uses and side effects may exist but further research is necessary to determine the exact properties and effects of use.

General: Holy Basil is native to India and is cultivated elsewhere. It is considered an invasive weed in some areas. It is easily propagated by seed and will self-seed readily.

Holy Basil leaves have been used as an insect repellant. The leaves are used as a seasoning in a variety of dishes or as a tea. The leaves are harvested and the oils extracted or the leaf, seed, and stem are harvested, dried, and powdered for use in traditional supplements.

Honeysuckle, Chevrefeuille, Goat's Leaf, Honey Suckle, Suikazura, Woodbine

Botanical Name:
Lonicera periclymenum

Properties:
Antibacterial, Anti-inflammatory, Antispasmodic, Antiviral, Antiseptic, Cathartic, Diuretic, Emetic, Emollient, Expectorant, Febrifuge, Laxative, Sedative, Vulnerary

Traditional Uses:
Honeysuckle is used as a traditional infusion to reduce bronchial inflammation and act to reduce the duration and severity of common respiratory infections like colds, and influenza.

Parts Used:
Flower, Leaf, Seed

Side Effects:
Honeysuckle is not recommended for use by women who are pregnant or nursing.

Additional uses and side effects may exist but further research is necessary to determine the exact properties and effects of use.

General:
Honeysuckle is a common bush or climbing vine cultivated in many regions of the world as a Honeysuckle is a common bush or climbing vine cultivated in many regions of the world as a fragrant ornamental. Hardy to zone 5, it is not particular regarding soil composition or sun but does prefer consistent moisture. Honeysuckle can be propagated by seeds sown out as soon as they are ripe, cuttings taken in mid summer or layering.

Honeysuckle flowers yield sweet, sugary nectar or the oils are extracted for use in perfumery. The fruits are eaten as a cooked food while the flowers have been used as an aromatic tea.

Honeysuckle leaf, seed, and flower are harvested, dried, and powdered for use in traditional supplement infusions.

Honeysuckle – Japanese, Japanese Honeysuckle

Botanical Name:
Lonicera japonica

Properties:

Antibacterial, Anti-inflammatory, Antimicrobial, Antispasmodic, Antiviral, Astringent, Depurative, Diuretic, Febrifuge, Hypotensive

Traditional Use:
Japanese Honeysuckle flowers & leaves are broad spectrum antimicrobials used in traditional supplements to treat a variety of bacterial and viral infectious agents including a numerous influenza strains, pseudomonas aeruginosa, salmonella typhi, staphylococcus aureus and streptococcus pneumoniae.

Part Used:
Bark, Flower, Leaf

Side Effects:
Japanese Honeysuckle is not recommended for use by women who are pregnant or nursing.

Additional uses and side effects may exist but further research is necessary to determine the exact properties and effects of use.

General:
Japanese Honeysuckle is native to Asia and is commonly cultivated in many regions of the world as a fragrant and ornamental. Hardy to zone 4, it is not particular regarding soil composition but does prefer full or partial sun and consistent moisture. It can be propagated by seeds sown out as soon as they are ripe, cuttings taken in the mid summer or by layering in the fall.

Japanese Honeysuckle has been used in Chinese supplements for thousands of years. The leaves are harvested and eaten as a cooked vegetable while the flowers are used as a sweet syrup. The bark, flower, and leaves are harvested at the end of the growing season, dried, and powdered for use in traditional topical and infusion preparations.

Hyssop, Curdukotu, Jufa, Ysop

Botanical Name:
Hyssopus officinalis

Properties:
Abortifacient, Anti-inflammatory, Antimicrobial, Antiseptic, Antispasmodic, Antiviral, Astringent, Carminative, Diaphoretic, Diuretic, Emmenagogue, Expectorant, Hypertensive, Nervine, Sedative, Vermifuge, Vulnerary

Traditional Use:
Hyssop has been used as a traditional supplement to reduce congestion in conditions like asthma, bronchitis, colds, influenza, and other lung infections and to reduce the duration and severity of any underlying infection.

The leaves and oils of the hyssop have antimicrobial properties that are traditionally used to combat topical and internal bacterial and viral infections.

Part Used:
Flower, Leaf, Oil

Side Effects:
Hyssop is not recommended for use by women who are pregnant or nursing.

Hyssop has been used as an abortifacient in some cultures.

Hyssop is not recommended for use in children's treatments.

Hyssop is not recommended for use by people with a history of seizures.

Additional uses and side effects may exist but further research is necessary to determine the exact properties and effects of use.

General:
Hyssop is native to the Mediterranean but is cultivated in the United States as an ornamental or for its oils. Hardy to zone 7, it prefers sandy to loamy soil, full sun, and consistent moisture. Hyssop can be propagated by seeds sown in the spring, cuttings taken in mid summer or division.

Hyssop oils are extracted through steam distillation for use in food, perfumery, aromatherapy, and traditional preparations. The flowers, leaves, and young shoots are eaten as a raw vegetable or flavoring additive. The whole plant, but especially the leaves are harvested during flowering, dried, and powdered for use in traditional supplemental infusions given throughout the day.

Immortelle, Shrubby Everlasting, Eternal Flower, Goldilocks, Sandy Everlasting, Strawflower, Yellow Chaste Weed

Botanical Name:
Helichrysum angustifolium

Properties:
Analgesic, Antibacterial, Anti-inflammatory, Antispasmodic, Antiviral, Cytophaylactic, Depurative, Diuretic, Expectorant, Hypoallergenic, Immunostimulant, Nervine

Traditional Use:
Immortelle has traditionally been used to alleviate constriction and excess congestion in conditions like asthma, bronchitis, colds, and influenza while acting to fight any bacteria or virus causing any related infection.

Immortelle has been used as a traditional supplement to help stimulate the immune system helping to prevent or shorten the duration of common infections.

Part Used:
Flower

Side Effects:
Immortelle is not recommended for use by women who are pregnant or nursing.

Immortelle is not recommended for use in children's treatments.

Immortelle is not recommended for use by people who have a blocked bile duct or gallstones.

Immortelle may cause an allergic reaction in some people.

Additional uses and side effects may exist but further research is necessary to determine the exact properties and effects of use.

General:
Immortelle is native to Europe and the United States. It prefers sandy or loamy soil, full or partial sunlight and consistent moisture. It is easily propagated by seeds direct sown as soon as they are ripe or by division of suckers in the spring.

The flowers are harvested as the buds begin to bloom. They are dried, powdered, and used in traditional supplement teas up to 3 times daily. Immortelle oil is steam distilled within 24 hours of harvesting the flower for use in topical and aromatherapy preparations.

Indigo – Wild, American Indigo, Baptista, False Indigo, Horsefly Weed, Indigo Broom, Rattlebush, Wild Indigo, Yellow Indigo

Botanical Name:
Baptisia tinctoria

Properties:
Adaptogen, Antibacterial, Antiseptic, Antiviral, Astringent, Cholagogue, Colorant, Emetic, Estrogenic, Febrifuge, Immunostimulant

Traditional Use:
Wild Indigo has been used as a traditional supplemental infusion to reduce the length and severity of infections of the upper respiratory tract including bronchitis, colds, and influenza.

Wild Indigo has been used as a traditional supplement to stimulate the immune system, help support antibody production, and ward off common infections.

Part Used:
Root

Side Effects:

Wild Indigo is not recommended for use by women who are pregnant or nursing.

Wild Indigo is not recommended for use in children's treatments.

Wild Indigo may cause skin irritation in some people.

Wild Indigo is not recommended for people with gastrointestinal disorders.

Overuse of Wild Indigo may cause diarrhea, difficulty breathing, increased heart rate, nausea, vomiting or even death.

Additional uses and side effects may exist but further research is necessary to determine the exact properties and effects of use.

General:
Wild Indigo is a perennial native to eastern North America. Hardy to zone 5, it prefers sandy or loamy soil and has the ability top add nitrogen back into nutritionally poor areas. It does require full sun and prefers consistent moisture. It can be propagated by seed sown out as soon as it is ripe and it self-seeds readily. Wild Indigo can also be propagated by division of larger clumps early in the growing season.

Wild Indigo is related to Dyer's Indigo and has smaller concentrations of blue toned colorant valued in dyeing and can be used in larger quantity to achieve the same tones. The young shoots are sometimes eaten as a vegetable.

Wild Indigo root is harvested, dried and powdered for use in traditional supplement infusions up to 3 times daily or in ointment preparations at a rate of 1:1 in 60% alcohol.

Juniper, Guinevere, Ginepro, Juniper Berries, Zimbro

Botanical Name:
Juniperus communis

Properties:

Abortifacient, Analgesic, Antibacterial, Antifungal, Anti-inflammatory, Antiseptic, Antispasmodic, Antiviral, Aphrodisiac, Arthritis, Astringent, Cancer, Carminative, Circulation, Depurative, Diaphoretic, Disinfectant, Diuretic, Emmenagogue, Hypotensive, Insect Repellant, Nervine, Rubefacient, Sedative, Tonic, Vermifuge

Traditional Use:
Juniper is used as an ingredient in disinfecting household cleaning products.

Juniper has been used as a traditional supplement to prevent or treat viral infections like herpes and influenza.

Juniper berries are traditionally used in steam treatments to help loosen and expel phlegm in congestive conditions like asthma, bronchitis, colds, influenza, and pneumonia and to shorten the duration of the infection.

Part Used:
Berry, Needles, Oil

Side Effects:
Juniper is not recommended for use by women who are pregnant or nursing.

Juniper berries are not recommended for use by women who suffer from heavy menstrual bleeding. They have been used as a dietary abortifacient in some cultures and are known to increase menstrual bleeding.

Juniper is not recommended for use by people who have diabetes, intestinal disorders, high blood pressure, or kidney disease.

Juniper may increase bleeding and is not recommended for use by those who have a bleeding disorder.

Overuse of Juniper may cause urine to smell like violets.

Overdose of Juniper can cause kidney irritation, blood in the urine, and potential liver damage.

Juniper oil is for external use only.

Additional uses and side effects may exist but further research is necessary to determine the exact properties and effects of use.

General:
Juniper is an evergreen shrub native to Africa, Asia, and Europe and has been naturalized to parts of North America. Hardy to zone 2, it is not particular regarding soil composition but does prefer full to partial sun. It prefers consistent moisture but will tolerate drought once established. Juniper can be propagated by seed but the hard seed coat may make germination difficult. Propagation from cuttings taken late in the year or by layering is more successful.

Juniper branches and extractions are used as part of traditional insect repelling preparations. The fruits are harvested in the fall and eaten raw or cooked as a flavoring in a variety of dishes. The seeds are roasted and used as a coffee substitute.

Juniper berries are harvested for use as a diet or tea supplement while the oils are extracted from the needles. Do not bruise or crush the berries until you are ready to use them.

Larch, Larix

Botanical Name:
Larix decidua

Properties:
Antibacterial, Antiseptic, Antiviral, Astringent, Binding Agent, Cholesterol, Diuretic, Emollient, Expectorant, Haemostatic, Immunostimulant, Laxative, Stabilizer, Starch, Vulnerary

Traditional Use:
Larch bark has traditionally been used to treat a tendency toward infection minimizing the likelihood of contracting common viral infections while acting to expand the bronchial passages and expel excess mucus in congestive conditions like asthma, bronchitis, colds, and influenza.

Larch is traditionally used to help boost the immune system and is frequently used as a prophylactic against common infections.

Part Used:
Outer Bark

Side Effects:
Larch is not recommended for use by women who are pregnant or nursing.

Larch is an immunostimulant and is not recommended for use by people with an immunoreactive disease like Multiple Sclerosis or Lupus.

Additional uses and side effects may exist but further research is necessary to determine the exact properties and effects of use.

General:
Larch is native to Europe and has been naturalized in North America. Hardy to zone 4, it prefers sandy to loamy soil, full sun, and moist to wet conditions. Larch can be propagated by seeds cold stored and then sown in the spring.

Larch wood resin is used to preserve wood and the wood itself is used in construction. The inner bark is eaten or dried and ground into flour. The bark is also harvested, dried, and powdered for use in traditional supplements.

Lavender

Botanical Name:
Lavandula angustifolia, Lavandula officinalis

Properties:
Analgesic, Antibacterial, Anti-inflammatory, Antifungal, Antioxidant, Antiseptic, Antispasmodic, Antiviral, Cancer, Colorant, Cardio-Tonic, Carminative, Deodorant, Diuretic, Emmenagogue, Hypotensive, Insect Repellant, Muscle Relaxant, Nervine, Sedative, Vermifuge

Traditional Use:
Lavender is traditionally included in topical applications and room sprays as an antiseptic to kill germs, reduce congestion, and ease constriction related to asthma, bronchitis, colds, and influenza.

Lavender oil has been used as a cleaning agent to kill bacterial, fungal, and viral infections.

Part Used:
Flower, Leaf, Stem

Side Effects:
Lavender is not recommended for use by women who are pregnant or nursing.

There have been reports that topical use of lavender oil can cause breast growth in boys, men, and young women.

Lavender may cause changes in appetite, constipation, headaches, and drowsiness in some people.

Lavender can cause skin irritation in some people.

Lavender is not recommended for use with anti-anxiety, antidepressants, antihistamines, or sedatives.

Overuse of lavender oil for internal supplements can be toxic if taken by mouth. Oils are for external use only. The leaves have been ingested.

Additional uses and side effects may exist but further research is necessary to determine the exact properties and effects of use.

General:
Lavender is native to the Mediterranean and was used in supplements and ceremonial treatments in ancient Egypt, Greece, and Rome. Hardy to zone 5, it is cultivated worldwide for use as a traditional aromatherapy, supplement tea, or extract. Lavender is not particular regarding soil composition but does prefer full sun, well-drained soil, and consistent

moisture. It can be propagated by seed sown out in the spring or by cuttings taken in the mid-summer with a heel of the previous year's growth.

Lavender essential oil is used in a variety of cosmetic, perfumery, and aromatherapy recipes. The oil is used as an insect repellant ingredient. The flowers are harvested as soon as the blooms begin to fade and the oils steam extracted. The flower, leaf, and stem are harvested for use fresh or dried and powdered for use in traditional topical, aromatherapy and supplemental treatments.

Lemon, Lemon Oil

Botanical Name:
Citrus limonum

Properties:
Adaptogen, Antibacterial, Anti-inflammatory, Antimicrobial, Antioxidant, Antiviral, Astringent, Carminative, Diuretic, Homeostatic, Immunostimulant, Rubefacient, Stimulant

Traditional Use:
Lemon oil has natural antibacterial properties and a refreshing scent that makes it a good choice in natural house cleaning products.

Lemon oil has been used as an antibacterial & antiviral supplement and topical preparation to treat infections.

Lemon is high in vitamin C and is traditionally used in immunity building programs helping the body to fight off infections.

Lemon is traditionally included in vapor treatments to disinfect the air and provide an uplifting and refreshing scent.

Part Used:
Juice, Rind - Oil

Side Effects:

Lemon is not recommended for use beyond dietary by women who are pregnant or nursing.

Lemon oil is phototoxic increasing the effect of sunlight on the skin.

Lemon oil should be diluted when using in any remedy as it may irritate the skin.

Additional uses and side effects may exist but further research is necessary to determine the exact properties and effects of use.

General:
Lemon is native to India but has been cultivated in other parts of the world. Hardy to zone 9, it prefers loamy or heavy, well-drained soils with full sun and consistent moisture. Lemon can be propagated by seed, rinsed and sown as soon as it is ripe or by cuttings taken in the mid-summer.

Lemon rind oils are used as a flavoring, perfume component, and household cleaner. Lemon seed oil has been used in soap making and the oils from the leaves are commonly called petitgrain oil in aromatherapy though the Bitter Orange is the source of true petitgrain. Lemon juice is used as a cleaning and bleaching product.

Lemon fruits are eaten raw, cooked, or as a beverage. Lemon oil is extracted from the rind or seed for use in traditional and topical preparations. It is harvested for use in culinary, supplement, cosmetic, and cleaning recipes.

Lemon Balm, Balm Dropsy Plant, Honey Plan, Melissa, Sweet Balm, Sweet Mary, Toronjil

Botanical Name:
Melissa officinalis

Properties:
Anodyne, Antibacterial, Antidepressant, Antihistamine, Antioxidant, Antispasmodic, Antiviral, Cardiac, Carminative, Diaphoretic, Diaphoretic,

Digestive, Emmenagogue, Febrifuge, Hypotensive, Hypothyroid, Insect Repellant, Nervine, Sedative, Styptic, Tonic

Traditional Use:
Lemon balm has been included in a European commercial preparation and traditional ointments to reduce the severity and duration of cold sore and herpes sore outbreaks.

Lemon Balm tea has antiviral properties. It has traditionally been used to induce sweating and reduce the severity and duration of common viral infections like influenza.

Part Used:
Flower, Leaf

Side Effects:
Lemon Balm is not recommended for use by women who are pregnant or nursing.

Lemon Balm may cause abdominal pain, dizziness, nausea, vomiting, and wheezing in some people.

Lemon Balm may cause an allergic reaction in some people.

Lemon balm has a sedative action and users should use not operate heavy machinery or drive while using Lemon Balm.

Additional uses and side effects may exist but further research is necessary to determine the exact properties and effects of use.

General:
Lemon Balm is a perennial native to the Mediterranean and Asia but is cultivated elsewhere. Hardy to zone 4, Lemon Balm grows easily from cuttings, division, or seed and is adaptable to a wide variety of soils, sun, and water conditions. Some people consider lemon balm to be an invasive plant.

Lemon Balm is grown both indoors and outdoors to help repel insects or used as part of a topical insect repellant preparation.   Lemon balm is harvested before blooming, separated into parts for use fresh or dried. Lemon Balm is traditionally given as a supplement tea up to 4 times daily. Fresh tea is more potent than dried since the oils tend to be diminished during the drying process. The oils are extracted by steam distillation for use as a traditional inhalant therapy.

Licorice, Black Sugar, Gan-Cao, Licorice, Licorice Root, Liquorice, Sweet Root

Botanical Name: Glycyrrhiza glabra

Properties: Antibacterial, Antifungal, Antiinflammatory, Antiperspirant, Antitussive, Antiviral, Cancer, Deodorant, Depurative, Demulcent, Detoxification, Diuretic, Emollient, Expectorant, Laxative, Liver Function, Phytoestrogen, Tonic

Traditional Use: Licorice root has traditionally been used to soothe the mucus membranes and expel excess mucus in congestive conditions like asthma, bronchitis, colds, and influenza while acting to treat any underlying infection.

Licorice root is used as a traditional supplement to speed the healing of many disorders of the gastrointestinal tract including heartburn, IBS, intestinal ulcers, gastric reflux, and duodenal, gastric, and peptic ulcers and to treat any underlying viral or bacterial infection.

Part Used: Root

Side Effects: Licorice root is not recommended for use by women who are pregnant or nursing.

Licorice root is not recommended for use in children's treatments.

Licorice root containing glycyrrhizin can cause high blood pressure, elevated sodium levels, low potassium levels, and water retention in some people.

Licorice root is not recommended for long-term use.

Licorice is not recommended for use with diuretics, corticosteroids, or other medicines that reduce the body's potassium levels.

Licorice is not recommended for use by those with heart disease or high blood pressure.

Licorice root can affect the body's levels of cortisole.

Licorice root might affect estrogen and is not recommended for use by women who have an estrogen related condition.

Licorice root can cause fatigue, headache, menstrual irregularity, water retention and a decrease of sexual function and interest.

Additional uses and side effects may exist but further research is necessary to determine the exact properties and effects of use.

General: Licorice root is native to Asia, Greece, and Turkey and has a long history of supplement use in both eastern and western medicine. Hardy to zone 8, it prefers sandy or loamy soil, full or partial sunlight and consistent moisture. Licorice can grow in poor quality soils and is known to fix nitrogen back into the soil. It can be propagated by seeds that are soaked in warm water and then sown in a controlled environment or by division or the root buds in the spring.

The root is harvested when it is mature, peeled, dried, and powdered or made in to an extract for use in topical preparations, traditional supplements, or culinary products. Licorice root sometimes has glycyrrhizin removed. Licorice with glycyrrhizin removed will not have the same supplemental benefits.

Lomatium, Indian Carrot

Botanical Name:
Lomatium dissecta

Properties:

Antibacterial, Antifungal, Antimicrobial, Antiviral, Expectorant, Stimulant

Traditional Use:
Lomatium is a stimulating expectorant, antibacterial and antiviral that is traditionally used to relieve congestion associated with conditions like asthma, bronchitis, colds, influenza, and pneumonia while helping to shorten the duration and lessen the severity of conditions caused by an infection.

Lomatium has traditionally been used to combat infection including viral infections like influenza, bacterial infections like streptococcus, and fungal infections like athlete's foot.

Lomatium has been added to cleaning preparations to kill surface bacteria, fungus, and viruses.

Part Used:
Resin, Root

Side Effects:
Lomatium is not recommended for use by women who are pregnant or nursing.

Lomatium may cause a severe allergic skin reaction in some people.

Additional uses and side effects may exist but further research is necessary to determine the exact properties and effects of use.

General:
Lomatium is native to North America where the roots are harvested, dried, and powdered for use as a traditional supplement.

Maritime Pine

Botanical Name:
Pinus pinaster

Properties:

Adoptogenic, Analgesic, Antihistamine, Antioxidant, Antiseptic, Antiviral, Colorant, Diuretic, Herbicide, Hypoglycemic, Hypotensive, Immunity, Rubefacient, Stimulant, Vasodilator, Vermifuge

Traditional Use:
Maritime Pine has traditionally been used to stimulate the immune system to minimize the likelihood of infection.

Maritime Pine has been used in traditional preparations to treat viral infections like influenza.

Part Used:
Bark

Side Effects:
Maritime Pine is not recommended for use by women who are pregnant or nursing.

Maritime Pine is not recommended for use by people who have an autoimmune disorder like lupus or multiple sclerosis.

Maritime Pine may cause dizziness, headaches, and gastro-intestinal upset.

Maritime Pine may lower blood sugar.

Maritime Pine may lower blood pressure.

Maritime Pine bark or dust may cause contact dermatitis in some people.

Additional uses and side effects may exist but further research is necessary to determine the exact properties and effects of use.

General:
Maritime Pine is native to Africa and Europe but is cultivated in other regions for use in commercial and traditional supplement preparations. Hardy to zone 8, it is not particular regarding soil composition but does prefer full sun and consistent moisture. It can be propagated by seed sown out as soon as it is ripe or by cuttings taken from young trees during the summer months.

Maritime Pine needles yield a greenish toned dye product and a fluid extracted from the needles has been used as an herbicide that helps to halt the germination of plants. The resin from the tree is used to make turpentine. Maritime Pine seed is eaten as a raw or cooked food or ground for use as flour. The bark is used in hundreds of patented supplements around the world. The bark is harvested, dried, and powdered or the resin extracted for use in traditional or commercial topical and supplemental preparations.

Mountain Lovage, Bear Root, Chuchpate, Colorado Cough Root, Indian Parsley, Mountain Carrot, Osha, Porters Licorice, Wild Celery Root

Botanical Name:
Ligusticum porteri

Properties:
Antibacterial, Antispasmodic, Antiviral, Astringent, Emmenagogue, Expectorant

Traditional Uses:
Mountain Lovage is used as a traditional supplement to reduce inflammation and congestion associated with conditions like bronchitis, colds, influenza, and pneumonia and to help shorten the severity and duration of respiratory infection.

Mountain Lovage has been used to reduce the number and severity of herpes outbreaks.

Parts Used:
Root

Side Effects:
Mountain Lovage is not recommended for use by women who are pregnant or nursing.

Mountain Lovage is not recommended for use in children's treatments, by people who have kidney disease, liver disease, and should only be used after consultation with a qualified herbalist or physician.

Additional uses and side effects may exist but further research is necessary to determine the exact properties and effects of use.

General:
Wild Lovage is native to North America where it has been used as a traditional supplement for hundreds of years. The root and seed are harvested and the oils extracted or dried & powdered for use as a traditional supplement.

Mullein, Adam's Flannel, Beggar's Blanket, Blanket Herb, Candleflower, Candlewick, Duffle, Feltwort, Flannel Leaf, Flannelflower, Great Mullein, Woolen

Botanical Name:
Verbascum thapsus

Properties:
Anodyne, Antibacterial, Anticoagulant, Anti-inflammatory, Antimicrobial, Antiseptic, Astringent, Antiviral, Astringent, Colorant, Demulcent, Diuretic, Emollient, Expectorant, Immunostimulant, Narcotic, Sedative, Vulnerary

Traditional Use:
Mullein smoke or tea is traditionally used to treat constriction, cough, and congestion associated with asthma, bronchitis, colds, influenza, and pneumonia while acting to treat the underlying infection.

Mullein is used as a traditional supplement to shorten the length and severity viral infections including the common cold and influenza.

Part Used:
Leaf, Flower, Root

Side Effects:

Mullein is not recommended for use by women who are pregnant or nursing.

Mullein may interfere with the body's clotting ability and is not recommended for use without the advice of a qualified herbalist or physician.

Additional uses and side effects may exist but further research is necessary to determine the exact properties and effects of use.

General:
Mullein is native to Africa, Asia, and Europe but has been naturalized to North America where it is considered an invasive weed by some. Hardy to zone 3, it is not particular regarding soil composition or moisture but does require full sun. Mullein can be found growing wild in untended areas or propagated by seeds sown out in the spring.

The whole Mullein plant yields a yellow to green colorant used as a culinary or textile dye. Mullein flowers yield a yellow toned colorant used as a textile dye or hair colorant. The leaves are used to make a bland aromatic tea while the leaves and flowers make a sweeter tea. The leaf, flower, and root are harvested at the beginning of the flowering season, dried, and powdered for use in traditional supplement tea preparations.

Myrrh
Botanical Name: Commiphora myrrha

Properties: Anodyne, Antibacterial, Antifungal, Antimicrobial, Anti-inflammatory, Antiseptic, Astringent, Carminative, Emmenagogue, Expectorant, Hypoglycemic, Insect Repellant, Pulmonary Stimulant, Sedative, Tonic, Vulnerary

Traditional Use: Myrrh resin is traditionally used as a topical preparation to treat infection and speed healing in skin ulcers, cold sores, & canker sores.

Myrrh has antibacterial, antifungal, antiseptic, and astringent action that make it a traditional ingredient in mouthwashes, skin washes, and soaks for cleansing and treatments of bacterial infections, viral infections, and fungal diseases like athlete's foot and thrush.

Part Used: Resin

Side Effects: Myrrh is not recommended for use by women who are pregnant or nursing.

Overuse of Myrrh can cause nausea or vomiting.

Myrrh may affect the menstrual cycles in some women.

Individuals with diabetes should consult with a qualified herbalist or physician before using myrrh as it may affect blood sugar.

Additional uses and side effects may exist but further research is necessary to determine the exact properties and effects of use.

General: Myrrh is native to the Mediterranean but is cultivated in other regions where the resin is harvested during the summer months for use in perfumery and traditional supplements. The bark is wounded to cause the formation of oily resin that is harvested and the oils extracted by steam distillation.

Myrtle, Common Myrtle, Saharan Myrtle
Botanical Name: Myrtus communis

Properties: Antibacterial, Antibiotic, Antimicrobial, Antiseptic, Antiviral, Astringent, Cardiac, Carminative, Haemostatic, Rubefacient, Stimulant, Sedative, Tonic, Vermifuge

Traditional Use: An infusion of Myrtle has traditionally been used as a stimulating expectorant to help alleviate the congestion and constriction associated with respiratory ailments like asthma, bronchitis, colds, influenza, pneumonia and whooping cough and since myrtle has strong antibiotic properties it aids in reducing the length of the associated infection.

Part Used: Branch, Leaf, Twig

Side Effects: Myrtle is not recommended for use by women who are pregnant or nursing.

Additional uses and side effects may exist but further research is necessary to determine the exact properties and effects of use.

General: Myrtle is native to Asia but cultivated in other regions. Hardy to zone 8, it is not particular regarding soil composition but does prefer full sun and consistent moisture. Myrtle can be propagated by seeds soaked and sown in the spring, cuttings taken in mid summer or layering.

The aerial parts of the plant yield an essential oil used in perfumery, soap making, and natural care products. Myrtle fruits are eaten raw or cooked, the leaves are used as a flavoring, and the whole plant is harvested during the summer, dried, and powdered for use in traditional supplement infusions taken up to 3 times daily.

Neem, Arishtha, Beard Tree, Holy Tree, Indian Lilac, Margosa
Botanical Name: Azadirachta indica

Properties: Antibacterial, Antifungal, Anti-inflammatory, Contraceptive, Detoxifier, Emollient, Hypoglycemic, Immunostimulant, Insect Repellant, Purgative, Tonic, Vermifuge, Viral Infection

Traditional Use: Neem bark has been used as a traditional supplement to stimulate the immune system and help ward off infections or slow the progress of conditions like AIDS.

Neem has traditionally been used as a topical preparation to reduce infection while speeding healing of skin sores, ulcers, and wounds.

Neem oil and Neem leaf tea is used as a topical preparation and cleaning agent against a variety of viral infections like herpes, shingles, and influenza.

Part Used: Bark, Leaf, Seed Nut Oil

Side Effects: Neem is not recommended for use by women who are pregnant or nursing.

Neem is not recommended for use in children's treatments.

Neem is for external use only.

Neem is not recommended for use by people with an autoimmune disease like Multiple Sclerosis and Lupus.

Neem may lower blood sugar.

Large doses of Neem Oil can be toxic if taken internally.

Overuse of Neem may cause diarrhea, drowsiness, loss of consciousness, coma, and even death.

Additional uses and side effects may exist but further research is necessary to determine the exact properties and effects of use.

General: Neem is native to the tropical regions of Africa and Asia where all parts of the tree are harvested. Neem is hardy to zone 9 and has been grown as a container tree in other climates. It prefers a very high quality soil but is accepting of a wide ranger of soil composition. It can be propagated by seed. It requires well-drained soil and consistent watering.

The shoots & flowers of the Neem tree are harvested as a vegetable, the gum is used as a thickening agent, and the stems are used as a tooth cleaning brush. The seeds are harvested and the oil steam extracted or the barks & leaves are harvested, dried, & powdered for use in traditional supplements & cleaning products.

Negrito, Bitterwood, Maruba, Paradise Tree

Botanical Name:
Simarouba glauca

Properties:

Analgesic, Antibacterial, Antifungal, Antimicrobial, Antiviral, Astringent, Cancer, Vermifuge

Traditional Use:
Negrito has been used as a household cleaner to neutralize bacteria, fungus, and viruses in the air and on hard or soft surfaces.

Negrito has been used as a traditional preparation to treat viral infections like herpes, shingles, and influenza.

Part Used:
Bark, Wood

Side Effects:
Negrito is not recommended for use by women who are pregnant or nursing.

Overuse of Negrito may cause nausea, perspiration, or vomiting.

Additional uses and side effects may exist but further research is necessary to determine the exact properties and effects of use.

General:
Negrito is a flowering tree native to Central America and southern North America, especially along the coastal hammocks of Florida. Negrito is not particular regarding soil composition but does prefer full to partial sun and moist to wet soil. It can be propagated by seed collected early in the spring, dried, and then sown indoors. If the seed coat is removed, the seeds can be germinated inside a plastic bag in the sun and then the young plants removed for final placement.

The seed are harvested and the oils extracted as food oil and the bark is harvested, dried, & powdered for use as a topical preparation or traditional decoction given at a rate of 6 ounces 2 times daily.

Nettle, Bichu, Stinging Nettle, Utica

Botanical Name:

Urtica dioica

Properties:
Analgesic, Anodyne, Anti-arthritic, Antifungal, Anti-inflammatory, Astringent, Colorant, Cancer, Depurative, Diuretic, Galactagogue, Hypoglycemic, Laxative, Immunostimulant, Nutritive, Tonic

Traditional Use:
Stinging Nettle has antiviral properties and is used as a traditional supplement to inhibit viruses including some types of influenza, RSV, CMV and HIV.

Part Used:
Leaf, Stem

Side Effects:
Stinging Nettle is not recommended for use by women who are pregnant or nursing.

Stinging Nettle may increase blood clotting or thinning depending on the age of the plant and is not recommended for use without the advice of a qualified herbalist or physician.

Stinging Nettle can cause an allergic reaction or skin irritation.

Stinging Nettle is not recommended for use by people with edema related to cardiac or renal function or who have kidney disease.

Stinging Nettle may lower blood sugar.

Stinging Nettle may lower blood pressure.

Stinging Nettle may interfere with preparations for diabetes, hypertension, antidepressants, and morphine based preparations.

Additional uses and side effects may exist but further research is necessary to determine the exact properties and effects of use.

General:

Nettle is a perennial native to Asia and Europe but has been naturalized throughout North America. Hardy to zone 3, it is not particular regarding soil composition but does prefer full or partial sun and consistent moisture. Stinging nettle is easily propagated by seed sown out in the spring and will self-sow readily if given its own place in the garden. It can also be propagated by division at any time during the growing season.

Nettle stems are used to make a strong twine or cloth. The entire plant can be used to create a natural colorant in shades of yellow, gold, and beige depending on the strength and age of the plant. Mordant – Alum   The leaves and stems yield a green toned colorant used as a traditional dye product.

The young leaves are eaten as a cooked vegetable and the whole plant is harvested during the flowering season, dried, and powdered for use as a topical preparation or in a traditional supplement tea up to 3 times daily.

Niauli Oil, Caje Oil, Huile, Paperbark
Botanical Name: Melaleuca viridiflora

Properties: Analgesic, Antibacterial, Anti-inflammatory, Antiseptic, Circulation, Expectorant, Insecticide, Nervine, Stimulant, Vermifuge, Vulnerary

Traditional Uses: Niauli oils are traditionally used in a vapor, spray, or household cleaner to disinfect the air and surfaces.

Niauli oil is used to reduce bronchial inflammation in congestive conditions like asthma, bronchitis, colds, and influenza and to help reduce the length and severity of infections like the common cold or influenza.

Parts Used: Leaf, Twigs - Oil

Side Effects: Niauli Oil is not recommended for use by women who are pregnant or nursing.

Niauli Oil is not recommended for use in children's treatments.

Niauli Oil may cause diarrhea, nausea, or vomiting.

Overuse of Niauli Oil may cause breathing problems, circulation problems, and low blood pressure.

Additional uses and side effects may exist but further research is necessary to determine the exact properties and effects of use.

General: Niauli Oil is extracted from the leaves of the Melaleuca viridiflora tree native to Australia. Do not confuse Niauli oil with Tea Tree oil or Cajuput oil that is taken from a different species of the Melaleuca plant.

The Melaleuca viridiflora tree is native to Australia where the bark is used as bedding, containers, and building shelter. The essential oil is extracted from young leaves and twigs for use in traditional supplement and disinfectant preparations.

Oak, Durmast Oak, English Oak, Pedunculate Oak, Sessile Oak, Stave Oak, Stone Oak, Tanner's Oak, White Oak

Botanical Name:
Quercus robur

Properties:
Anodyne, Anti-inflammatory, Antiviral, Astringent, Cancer, Depurative, Emmenagogue, Styptic

Traditional Use:
The astringent properties of oak bark make it a traditional tea ingredient for the treatment congestion, constriction, & cough associated with conditions like asthma, bronchitis, colds, influenza, and pneumonia while acting to shorten the duration or minimize the severity of the underlying infection.

Part Used:
Bark

Side Effects:

Oak Bark is not recommended for use by women who are pregnant or nursing.

Oak Bark is not recommended for use by people who have fever, heart disease, hypertonia, kidney problems, or liver problems.

Overuse of Oak bark may cause stomach problems, intestinal problems, kidney damage, or liver damage.

Additional uses and side effects may exist but further research is necessary to determine the exact properties and effects of use.

General:
Oak trees are found in many regions of the world where the bark is harvested, dried, powdered, and used in supplement teas and rinses.

Oregano, Dostenkraut, Mountain Mint, Origan, Wild Marjoram, Winter Marjoram, Wintersweet

Botanical Name:
Origanum vulgare

Properties:
Anodyne, Antibacterial, Antifungal, Antimicrobial, Antioxidant, Antiparasitic, Antispasmodic, Antiviral, Cancer, Carminative, Cox-2 Inhibitor, Diaphoretic, Emmenagogue, Expectorant, Immunostimulant, Nervine, Rubefacient, Sedative, Stimulant, Vermifuge

Traditional Use:
Oregano has been used in traditional supplements to reduce the inflammation of the bronchial passages and expel excess mucus in conditions like asthma, bronchitis, colds, and influenza while acting to reduce the duration and severity of the underlying infection.

Oregano is used as a traditional supplement to help stimulate the immune system and ward off common infections.

Oregano oil has illustrated an ability to inhibit bacteria, fungus and viruses and is traditionally used in antibacterial, antifungal, and antiviral treatments and cleaning products.

Part Used:
Leaf, Oil, Stem

Side Effects:
Oregano is not recommended for use beyond dietary by women who are pregnant or nursing.

Oregano may cause an allergic reaction in some people.

Oregano may irritate the skin.

Additional uses and side effects may exist but further research is necessary to determine the exact properties and effects of use.

General:
Oregano is cultivated worldwide for culinary use and harvested during the flowering season when the oils are extracted by steam distillation for use in traditional supplement preparations. Dried Oregano is used as a culinary seasoning but is typically not strong enough for use as a supplement.

Pau D'Arco, Taheebo

Botanical Name:
Tabebuia avellanedae

Properties:
Analgesic, Antibacterial, Anti-inflammatory, Antifungal, Antimicrobial, Antioxidant, Antiviral, Astringent, Cancer, Hypotensive, Immunostimulant, Laxative, Sedative, Tonic

Traditional Use:
Pau D'Arco has been used as a traditional supplement to stimulate the immune system and prevent bacterial, fungal, and viral infections.

Pau D'Arco is used traditionally to prevent or treat viral infections acting shorten the length & severity of common infections like colds & influenza.

Part Used:
Inner Bark

Side Effects:
Pau D'Arco is not recommended for use by women who are pregnant or nursing.

Pau D'Arco may lower blood pressure.

Additional uses and side effects may exist but further research is necessary to determine the exact properties and effects of use.

General:
Pau D'Arco is a canopy tree native to the forests of Central and South America but has been naturalized to the southern parts of the United States. The bark has been harvested for thousands of years for use as a traditional supplement. Pau D'Arco is traditionally harvested, dried, shredded, and boiled for no less than 15 minutes prior to use as a traditional supplement.

Peppermint, Black Peppermint, Bo He, Brandy Mint, Lamb Mint, Mentha, Mint, Mint Balm, Sentebon, White Peppermint

Botanical Name:
Mentha x piperita officinalis, Mentha x piperita vulgaris

Properties:
Abortifacient, Adaptogen, Analgesic, Anodyne, Antibacterial, Antifungal, Antioxidant, Antispasmodic, Antiseptic, Antiviral, Astringent, Cancer, Cardiac, Carminative, Colorant, Cephalic, Cholagogue, Diaphoretic, Emmenagogue, Expectorant, Febrifuge, Hepatic, Insect Repellant, Muscle Relaxant, Nervine, Tonic, Vasoconstrictor, Vasodilator, Vermifuge

Traditional Use:

Peppermint is used as a traditional supplement to alleviate constriction and congestion associated with conditions like asthma, bronchitis, colds, influenza while acting to minimize the severity and duration of associated viral infection.

Peppermint tea is traditionally used to stimulate the immune system & combat infectious agents. It has been used to help reduce the length of common infections when used as soon as symptoms appear.

Part Used:
Leaf, Oil

Side Effects:
Peppermint is not recommended for use beyond dietary by women who are pregnant or nursing.

High amounts of Peppermint have been as an abortifacient in some cultures.

Peppermint can cause headache, heartburn, nausea, and mouth sores in some people.

Peppermint may cause an allergic reaction in some people.

Peppermint oil may irritate the eyes, nose, or gastro-intestinal tract.

Do not ingest peppermint oil. Peppermint oil is for topical use only unless special coated tablets are used for delivery.

Additional uses and side effects may exist but further research is necessary to determine the exact properties and effects of use.

General:
Peppermint is a cross between water mint and spearmint native to the Mediterranean but naturalized throughout much of the world. Hardy to zone 3, peppermint is a hardy perennial that spreads rapidly by runner in nearly any soil, sun, and water conditions and may become an invasive weed.

The leaves are eaten raw or cooked and have been used as a flavoring in a variety of beverage, culinary, and confectionary recipes. The whole plant is harvested before flowering and the essential oil extracted by steam distillation. The essential oil of peppermint is added to topical preparations. Peppermint leaves are traditionally used in a tea or powder form.

Pine – Scots, Dwarf Pine, Monterey Pine, Pine, Scots Fir, Scots Pine, Swiss Mountain Pine

Botanical Name:
Pinus sylvestris

Properties:
Analgesic, Anodyne, Antibacterial, Anti-inflammatory, Antiseptic, Antiviral, Appetite Depressant, Cancer, Colorant, Depurative, Diuretic, Expectorant, Rubefacient, Nervine, Vermifuge

Traditional Use:
Pine needles are traditionally used to reduce inflammation and congestion in respiratory disorders like asthma, bronchitis, colds, and stuffy nose while acting as a respiratory antiseptic to help shorten the duration of common infections like colds and influenza.

Pine oil is traditionally used in household cleaning products to help reduce bacteria & viruses and to treat parasitic infestations like bedbugs or scabies.

Part Used:
Needles, Oil, Resin

Side Effects:
Pine is not recommended for use by women who are pregnant or nursing.

Pine may cause an allergic reaction or skin irritation.

Additional uses and side effects may exist but further research is necessary to determine the exact properties and effects of use.

General:

Scots Pine is native to Asia & Europe and has been naturalized to North America. Hardy to zone 2, it prefers sandy to loamy soil but is not particular regarding soil nutrition. It prefers full or partial sun and consistent moisture. It is propagated by seed sown out as soon as it is ripe or by cuttings of young trees taken in the spring. Removing the needles form the branches to be cut a month prior to taking the cuttings sometimes helps with propagation.

Pinecones yield a brown to tan colorant used as a textile dye product and the needles yield a green toned dye. The resin is used to make turpentine and the pitch taken from the resin can be used as to waterproof wood and fabric. The inner bark is used to make rope and the roots are used as a candle substitute. The wood is used in furniture making and other woodcraft or to make paper. The inner bark has been dried and ground into flour and the resin can be distilled into a vanilla like flavoring.

The needles are harvested for use in traditional supplements or the oils steam extracted for use in topical, supplement, or inhalant preparations.

Poke Root, Indian Poke

Botanical Name:
Phytolacca acinosa

Properties:
Antiasthmatic, Antibacterial, Antifungal, Anti-inflammatory, Antitussive, Antiviral, Diuretic, Emetic, Expectorant, Laxative, Vermifuge

Traditional Uses:
Poke is being investigated for its potential benefit as a broad-spectrum antiviral and antibacterial and is considered potentially useful in treatments and preventatives for mutating viral infections. All parts of the plant are considered toxic and poke should only be used under the supervision of a qualified herbalist or physician.

Parts Used:
Root

Side Effects:
Poke is not recommended for use by women who are pregnant or nursing.

The entire poke plant may contain toxic compounds and should only be used under the supervision of a qualified herbalist or physician.

Additional uses and side effects may exist but further research is necessary to determine the exact properties and effects of use.

General:
Poke is native to eastern Asia and has naturalized in other parts of the world including North America. Hardy to zone 7, it is not particular regarding soil composition but prefers full to partial sun and consistent moisture. Poke can be propagated by seed sown in the spring or division of the clump early in the growing season.

Poke leaves, shoots, and root have traditionally been eaten as a cooked vegetable but some reports indicate they may contain toxic compounds. The fruits yield a red toned colorant traditionally used as an ink. The root is harvested in the fall, dried, and powdered for use in traditional preparations.

Pomegranate, Dadima

Botanical Name:
Punica granatum

Properties:
Antibacterial, Antioxidant, Antiviral, Astringent, Cardio-tonic, Colorant, Demulcent, Emmenagogue, Immunostimulant, Vermifuge

Traditional Use:
Pomegranate bark extracts are traditionally used to treat bacterial and viral infections.

Pomegranate bark extract is used as a traditional as part of household vapor and spray disinfecting preparations.

Part Used:
Bark, Fruit, Oil, Rind, Seed

Side Effects:
Pomegranate is not recommended for use by women who are pregnant or nursing.

Pomegranate bark extracts are very toxic. Do not use bark extracts.

Pomegranate may cause an allergic reaction in some people.

Overuse of Pomegranate may cause dizziness, gastric upset, vomiting, vision disorders, or even death.

Additional uses and side effects may exist but further research is necessary to determine the exact properties and effects of use.

General:
Pomegranate is native to Africa, China, and India and has been naturalized to parts of California and Arizona. Hardy to zone 9, it is not particular regarding soil composition or moisture but does prefer full sun. Pomegranate is easily propagated by seed, mature cuttings, layering, or by division of the suckers.

The dried rind of the pomegranate fruit produces colors ranging from deep yellow to greenish-yellow tones. The age of the fruit affects the final color of the dye with the less ripe fruits containing more green tones used in textile dyeing. Iron mordant gives a deep mossy green color. The flowers and unripe fruit rind yield a red to reddish black toned colorant used in cosmetics, textile dying, and ink. The root bark yields a deep black colorant with high tannins giving it the ability to act as a self-mordant.

Pomegranate yields a durable, yellow toned wood used in small woodcraft projects. Pomegranate fruits are eaten as a raw food and the juice is used raw or in the creation of soups, jellies, and sauces. Fresh seeds are eaten raw and the leaves are dried for use as a seasoning or eaten as a cooked vegetable.

Pomegranate has been harvested for use in traditional supplements for thousands of years. The bark, fruit, oils, rind, and seeds are all used in traditional preparations.

Purslane, Ma Chi Xian, Pigweed, Pursley

Botanical Name: Portulaca oleracea

Properties: Antibacterial, Antibiotic, Anticoagulant, Anti-inflammatory, Astringent, Cholesterol, Depurative, Diuretic, Febrifuge, Hypotensive, Vermifuge, Vulnerary

Traditional Use: Purslane is rich in omega 3 fatty acids and has been used as part of a traditional dietary treatment plan to stimulate immunity and help the body ward off common infections.

Part Used: Leaf

Side Effects: Purslane is not recommended for use by women who are pregnant or nursing.

Purslane may lower the body's ability to clot and is not recommended for use by people who are taking a blood thinning medication or who have a bleeding disorder.

Purslane may lower blood pressure.

Additional uses and side effects may exist but further research is necessary to determine the exact properties and effects of use.

General: Purslane is a succulent native to Asia and southern Europe but it has been naturalized to southern North America. It is considered an invasive weed in some regions but cultivated in others as a groundcover or nutritive leafy green vegetable. It Is not particular regarding soil composition but does prefer good drainage, full sun, and consistent moisture. It can be propagated by seed and will self-sow readily if given its own area in the garden.

The leaves and stems are eaten as a raw or cooked vegetable and the seeds are eaten raw or cooked or ground into flour. The plant has also been burnt and the ashes used as a salt substitute.

The leaves are harvested and used fresh or dried as a traditional supplement.

Ravensara, Clove Nutmeg

Botanical Name:
Ravensara aromatica

Properties:
Antibacterial, Antifungal, Antiseptic, Antiviral, Expectorant

Traditional Use:
Ravensara is used in air inhalants and traditional supplements to alleviate the congestion associated with conditions like asthma, bronchitis, colds, influenza, and pneumonia and to help fight infection and shorten the length and severity of common respiratory infections.

Ravensara oils are traditionally used in vapor therapy and household cleaners to reduce bacterial, fungal, and viral infectious agents.

Part Used:
Bark – Leaf – Oil

Side Effects:
Ravensara is not recommended for use by women who are pregnant or nursing.

Additional uses and side effects may exist but further research is necessary to determine the exact properties and effects of use.

General:
Ravensara is native to Madagascar and cultivated elsewhere for the essential oils extracted from the bark & leaves. The oils are extracted

through steam distillation and used in topical and aromatherapy preparations.

Red Mangrove

Botanical Name:
Rhizophora mangle

Properties:
Anti-inflammatory, Anti-ulcer, Antiviral, Astringent, Febrifuge, Gastro-Protective, Immunostimulant

Traditional Use:
Red Mangrove has been used as a traditional medicinal to shorten the severity and duration of infections like the common cold and influenza.

Part Used:
Bark, Leaf

Side Effects:
Red Mangrove is not recommended for use by women who are pregnant or nursing.

Additional uses and side effects may exist but further research is necessary to determine the exact properties and effects of use.

General:
Red Mangrove is a small tree native to the coastal regions of India where the bark and leaves are harvested for use in traditional treatments.

Rosemary, Old Man, Romarin, Romero, Rusmari, Rusmary

Botanical Name: Rosmarinus officinalis

Properties: Analgesic, Antibacterial, Antifungal, Antiinflammatory, Antimicrobial, Antioxidant, Antiseptic, Antispasmodic, Antiviral, Arthritis,

Astringent, Cancer, Cardio-Tonic, Cephalic, Circulation, Colorant, Cox-2 Inhibitor, Diaphoretic, Digestive, Diuretic, Emmenagogue, Hepatic, Hypertensive, Insect Repellant, Muscle Relaxant, Nervine, Rubefacient, Stimulant, Vermifuge

Traditional Use:
Rosemary leaves are used as a traditional treatment for viral, fungal and bacterial infections of the skin.

The leaves are used as an air purification element especially in sick rooms where its antibacterial, antifungal and antiviral properties are considered effective.

Side Effects: Rosemary is not recommended for use beyond dietary by women who are pregnant or nursing.

Rosemary has been used as an abortifacient in some cultures.

Rosemary is not recommended for use in children's treatments.

Rosemary is not recommended for use by people who have epilepsy or a similar condition.

Rosemary is not recommended for use by people who have Crohn's disease, ulcerative colitis, or ulcers.

Rosemary oil is for external use only and can be toxic if taken internally.

Rosemary may affect diabetes, high blood pressure, or the effectiveness of medications to control blood pressure or diabetes,

Rosemary may cause an allergic reaction in some people.

Additional uses and side effects may exist but further research is necessary to determine the exact properties and effects of use.

General: Rosemary is an evergreen shrub or herb native to Asia but has been naturalized in much of the world as a garden shrub and a kitchen herb. Hardy to zone 6, it prefers sandy to loamy soil, full sun, and consistent moisture.

The young flowers, leaves, and shoots are eaten as a raw or cooked vegetable or dried for use as a seasoning.   The leaves and flowers yield a yellow toned colorant used in culinary, cosmetic and textile dying. The oils from the leaves and stems are used in perfumery and soap making. The leaves are used as an air purification element especially in sick rooms where its antibacterial, antifungal and antiviral properties are considered effective.

The leaves are harvested after flowering, dried in the sun and incorporated into supplement teas used up to 4 times a day or as a 1:5 tincture with 70% ethanol. The oils are extracted through steam distillation for use in soap making, cosmetics, aromatherapy and topical preparations.

Sage Brush

Botanical Name:
Artemisia tridentate

Properties:
Antibacterial, Antimicrobial, Antiseptic, Antiviral, Astringent, Colorant, Febrifuge, Sedative

Traditional Use:
Sage Brush has been used as a disinfectant household cleaner
Part Used:
Leaf

Side Effects:
Sage Brush is not recommended for use by women who are pregnant or nursing.

Additional uses and side effects may exist but further research is necessary to determine the exact properties and effects of use.

General:

Sage Brush is an evergreen shrub native to Central & North America and cultivated in other regions. The bark is harvested for making baskets & other woven products or as insulation. The seeds have been harvested for the popping effect they give when tossed into an open fire and the wood is used in construction and as a burning product. The leaves are harvested for use as a cooked vegetable or in traditional supplements.

Sandalwood, Anaditam, Chandran, Chandana, Safed Chandan, Sandal Tree, Santal, Tan Xiang, White Sandalwood, Yellow Sandalwood, Yellow Saunders

Botanical Name:
Santalum album

Properties:
Anodyne, Antibacterial, Antifungal, Antiseptic, Antispasmodic, Antiviral, Aphrodisiac, Astringent, Carminative, Diuretic, Emollient, Expectorant, Sedative

Traditional Use:
Sandalwood acts as an expectorant and antispasmodic making it a traditional component in reducing congestion in conditions like asthma, bronchitis, colds, influenza and in calming a dry, unproductive cough while acting to minimize the severity and duration of any underlying infection.

Part Used:
Wood - Oil

Side Effects:
Sandalwood is not recommended for use other than aromatic by women who are pregnant or nursing.

Overuse of Sandalwood oil may affect the kidneys.

Sandalwood may cause an allergic reaction. These reactions include skin irritation, gastrointestinal upset, itching, and nausea.

Additional uses and side effects may exist but further research is necessary to determine the exact properties and effects of use.

General:
Sandalwood oil is extracted from the inner wood of the sandalwood tree. Sandalwood is a semi-parasitic tropical tree that depends on other trees for nourishment during its early development. Sandalwood has been over-harvested and it is presently considered an endangered botanical species. The oils are extracted through steam distillation for use in perfumery, aromatherapy, and supplemental treatments.

Scarlet Pimpernel, Adder's Eye, Poor Man's Weatherglass, Red Chickweed, Shepherd's Barometer

Botanical Name:
Anagallis arvensis

Properties:
Abortifacient, Antibacterial, Antifungal, Anti-inflammatory, Antitussive, Antiviral, Cholagogue, Diaphoretic, Diuretic, Estrogenic, Expectorant, Narcotic, Nervine, Spermicidal, Stimulant, Vulnerary

Traditional Use:
Scarlet Pimpernel has traditionally been used to reduce congestion in conditions like asthma, bronchitis, colds, and influenza while acting to shorten the duration and severity of the underlying infection.

Scarlet Pimpernel has been used as a traditional antiviral to treat viruses like adenoviruses, herpes, and polio among others.

Part Used:
Flower, Leaf, Stem

Side Effects:
Scarlet Pimpernel is not recommended for use by women who are pregnant or nursing.

Scarlet Pimpernel has been used as abortifacient in some cultures.

Scarlet Pimpernel is not for long-term topical or internal use.

Scarlet Pimpernel can cause internal swelling.

Scarlet Pimpernel may contain estrogen like compounds and is not recommended for those with an estrogen sensitive disorder like cancer or fibroids.

Scarlet Pimpernel may act as a spermicidal and is not recommended for use by women or men who are trying to conceive.

Scarlet Pimpernel is not recommended for use without the advice of a qualified herbalist or physician.

Additional uses and side effects may exist but further research is necessary to determine the exact properties and effects of use.

General:
Scarlet Pimpernel is native to Asia, Europe, and North America. Hardy to zone 7, it is not particular regarding soil composition but does require full sun and consistent moisture. Scarlet Pimpernel is easily propagated by seed sown out in the spring and will self-sow readily if given its own place in the garden.

The leaves are eaten as a raw or cooked vegetable and the whole plant has been used as a soap substitute.

The flower, leaf, and stem are harvested, dried, and powdered for use in poultices or traditional supplements.

Siberian Ginseng, Ciwujia, Devil's Bush, Devil's Shrub, Eleuthero, Racine, Touch Me Not, Untouchable, Ussuri, Russian Root, Thorny Pepperbush, Wild Pepper, Wu Jia Pi

Botanical Name:
Eleutherococcus senticosus

Properties:
Adaptogen, Antibacterial, Antiviral, Circulation, Immunostimulant, Stimulant

Traditional Use:
Siberian Ginseng has traditionally been used to stimulate the immune system and reduce the length, number, and severity of viral infections including the common cold and influenza and is traditionally given as soon as symptoms start to appear with results expected within 2 days of starting treatment.

Siberian Ginseng is used as a traditional preventative and treatment to reduce the number, severity, and duration of viral infections including herpes simplex type 2.

Part Used:
Root

Side Effects:
Siberian Ginseng is not recommended for use by women who are pregnant or nursing.

Siberian Ginseng is not recommended for use by people with heart conditions as it may cause high blood pressure, increased heart rate, and irregular heartbeat.

Siberian Ginseng is not recommended for use by people with a hormone sensitive condition like endometriosis, fibroids, or cancer.

Siberian Ginseng is not recommended for use by people with mental conditions like bi-polar disorder, depression, and schizophrenia.

Siberian Ginseng may cause anxiety, muscle spasms, and increased depression in some people.

Siberian Ginseng may lower blood sugar.

Siberian Ginseng should not be combined with products that contain caffeine.

Additional uses and side effects may exist but further research is necessary to determine the exact properties and effects of use.

General:
Siberian Ginseng is a woodland shrub native to China, Korea, Japan, and Siberia that has adapted in many other regions of the world. Hardy to zone 3, it is not particular regarding soil composition but does prefer full or partial sun and consistent moisture. Siberian Ginseng can be propagated by seeds sown out as soon as they are ripe, cuttings taken in mid-summer, root cuttings taken in the winter, or by division of the suckers at the end of the dormant season.

Ginseng leaf and buds are eaten as a cooked vegetable and the dried leaves are used as a tea substitute. It is harvested for use as a supplement extract or dried for use as a powder supplement. The benefits of Siberian Ginseng are noted over a period of weeks and it is traditionally given daily for 3-4 weeks and then not at all for the next 2-4 weeks.

Spicebush, Benjamin Bush, Northern Spicebush, Wild Allspice

Botanical Name:
Lindera benzoin

Properties:
Antibacterial, Antiseptic, Antiviral, Astringent, Diaphoretic, Disinfectant, Febrifuge, Insect Repellant, Stimulant, Tonic, Vermifuge

Traditional Use:
Spice Bush bark and bark oils have traditionally been used as an air inhalant, spray cleaner, or infusion to disinfect sick rooms.

Spice Bush bark decoctions are used as a traditional treatment for bacterial and viral infections.

Part Used:
Bark, Leaf, Leaf Oil

Side Effects:

Spice Bush is not recommended for use by women who are pregnant or nursing.

Additional uses and side effects may exist but further research is necessary to determine the exact properties and effects of use.

General:
Spice Bush is native to North America where it can be found growing wild along streams and in swampy areas. Hardy to zone 5, it is not particular regarding soil composition but does require partial shade and constantly wet soils. Spice Bush can be propagated by seeds sown out as soon as they are ripe, air layering, or cuttings taken in the mid summer.

Spice Bush leaves and leaf oils have been used to repel insects and the twigs and bark yield mint-scented oil.

Spruce, Fir Tree, Spruce Fir, Norway Spruce

Botanical Name:
Picea abies

Properties:
Antibacterial, Antiseptic, Antiviral, Astringent, Febrifuge, Hyperemic, Rubefacient

Traditional Use:
Spruce oil has been approved in Europe for use as a treatment for bronchitis, colds, congestion, coughs, and fevers. Fir helps to reduce mucus production in the airways while acting as a mild antibacterial & antiviral.

Part Used:
Needles - Oil

Side Effects:
Spruce is not recommended for use by women who are pregnant or nursing.

Spruce is not recommended for individuals suffering from bronchial asthma as it may make symptoms worse.

Spruce should not be applied to broken skin or over large areas of skin.

Additional uses and side effects may exist but further research is necessary to determine the exact properties and effects of use.

General:
Spruce is an evergreen tree native to Europe but is cultivated in other regions of the world as an ornamental. Spruce oil is extracted from the branches and needles where it is traditionally taken as an infusion at a rate of 4 drops up to 3 times daily, an inhalant, or as an external ointment at a rate of 25% overall mixture.

St. John's Wort, Amber, Goatweed, Tipton Weed

Botanical Name:
Hypericum perforatum

Properties:
Abortifacient, Analgesic, Anodyne, Antibacterial, Ant-Inflammatory, Antidepressant, Antifungal, Antimicrobial, Antioxidant, Antiseptic, Antispasmodic, Antiviral, Astringent, Cholagogue, Colorant, Digestive, Diuretic, Expectorant, Nervine, Sedative, Stimulant, Vermifuge, Vulnerary

Traditional Use:
St. John's Wort tea and tinctures have traditionally been used to treat viral infections like herpes, influenza A, and parainfluenza.

Part Used:
Flower, Leaf

Side Effects:
St. John's Wort is not recommended for use by women who are pregnant or nursing.

St. John's Wort is not recommended for use by women who are trying to conceive.

St. John's Wort has been used as an abortifacient in some cultures.

St. John's Wort may cause skin irritation.

St. John's Wort is not recommended for use by people with Bipolar Disorder, Schizophrenia, or Severe Depression.

St. John's Wort may interfere with the function of a variety of supplement and prescription products.

St. John's Wort is not recommended for use by people who are on prescription antidepressants.

St. John's Wort may cause increased sensitivity to sunlight.

St. John's Wort may cause dizziness, dry mouth, fatigue, gastrointestinal upset, headache, and sexual dysfunction in some people.

Additional uses and side effects may exist but further research is necessary to determine the exact properties and effects of use.

General:
John's Wort is native to Africa, Asia, and Europe and is cultivated in other regions for supplemental purposes. Hardy to zone 3, it is not particular regarding soil composition but does prefer good drainage, full to partial sun and consistent moisture. It can be propagated by seeds sown out as soon as they are ripe or by division in the spring.

The flowering tops of the St. John's Wort are harvested during the flowering season, dried, and used in traditional supplement teas, extracts and in powdered form for both internal and topical applications.

Star Anise

Botanical Name:

Illicium verum

Properties:
Antibacterial, Antifungal, Antispasmodic, Antiviral, Carminative, Expectorant, Phytoestrogen, Relaxant, Stimulant

Traditional Use:
Star Anise contains the compound Oseltamivir, which is the primary ingredient in Tamiflu and has traditionally been used in medicinals to shorten the duration and severity of common infections like influenza.

Aromatherapy:
Cheering, Euphoric

Star Anise has a distinct anise-like aroma that blends well with citrus, lavender, and mint.

Part Used:
Fruit, Seed - Oil

Side Effects:
Star Anise is not recommended for use by women who are pregnant or nursing.

Star Anise is not recommended for use in children's treatments.

Star Anise is not recommended for use by people who have a hormone sensitive disorder like endometriosis, fibroids, or cancer.

Star Anise may cause an allergic reaction or skin irritation in some people.

Additional uses and side effects may exist but further research is necessary to determine the exact properties and effects of use.

General:
Star Anise is native to Asia and cultivated in other areas. Hardy to zone 8, it prefers sandy to loamy soil, full to partial sun and consistent moisture. Star Anise can be propagated by seed sown out in the spring, layering during the growing season, or cuttings taken in the late summer.

Star Anise bark is pounded and burnt for the scent and the fruit is used as a flavoring or harvested when nearly ripe used fresh, dried, or as an essential oil in traditional supplements.

Tamarind, Imlee, Tintiri

Botanical Name: Tamarindus indica

Properties: Antibacterial, Antifungal, Anti-inflammatory, Antimicrobial, Antiseptic, Digestive, Immunostimulant, Laxative, Vermifuge, Vulnerary

Traditional Use: Tamarind has traditionally been used to stimulate the immune system and to prevent common infections.

Part Used: Fruit, Seed

Side Effects: Tamarind is not recommended for use by women who are pregnant or nursing.

Additional uses and side effects may exist but further research is necessary to determine the exact properties and effects of use.

General: Tamarind is a large evergreen native to Africa and has been naturalized to North & South America where the fruit is harvested when ripe for use as a food. The oil is extracted from the seed through steam distillation for use in topical preparations, cosmetics, and supplements.

Tea, Black Tea, Chinese Tea, English Tea, Green Tea

Botanical Name:
Camellia sinensis

Properties:
Analgesic, Anti-inflammatory, Antioxidants, Antispasmodic, Antiviral, Appetite Depressant, Astringent, Cancer, Cardio-tonic, Colorant, Cox-2, Diuretic, Inhibitor, Hypoglycemic, Hypotensive, Nervine, Stimulant

Traditional Use:
Black tea is traditionally used as a gentle eyewash treatment for conjunctivitis and as a traditional wash to reduce inflammation, fight viral infection like herpes infection.

Part Used:
Leaves

Side Effects:
Tea is not recommended for use in women who are pregnant or nursing.

Tea is not recommended for use by people who have anemia, anxiety, bleeding disorders, diabetes, glaucoma, heart problems, high blood pressure, osteoporosis, or an overactive thyroid.

Tea is not recommended for use in women who have a hormone sensitive condition like endometriosis, fibroids, and cancer.

Overdose of tea may cause confusion, convulsions, diarrhea, dizziness, headache, heartburn, irregular heartbeat, nervousness, sleep problems, tremor, and vomiting.

Green tea contains compounds that may make anticoagulant drugs less effective.

Tea does contain caffeine and overuse may lead to anxiety, frequent urination, irritability, insomnia, restlessness, and upset stomach.

There have been reports of liver problems in some people taking a concentrated tea extract over an extended period.

Tea may be addictive.

Additional uses and side effects may exist but further research is necessary to determine the exact properties and effects of use.

General:

Tea is cultivated in many parts of the world as a commonly consumed beverage. Hardy to zone 8, it prefers sandy to loamy soils with good drainage, partial sun, and consistent moisture. Tea can be propagated by seeds sown out as soon as they are ripe or by cuttings taken at any time during the growing season.

Black, brown, and green teas come from the same plant and the difference in coloring is a result of a change in the way that the tea is handled during processing. The more extensive the handling, the darker the tea product and resulting colorant. Brown Tea is only partially fermented while Black Tea is fully fermented and Green Tea is not fermented.

Tea leaves yield an essential oil used in perfumery and as a culinary flavoring. The seeds yield oil used in manufacturing. Tea flower petals yield a greenish gray to black toned colorant used as a textile dye. The leaves yield a tan to deep brown toned colorant used as a culinary, cosmetic, or textile dye. The wood is used to make small woodcraft.

Tea is typically brewed and consumed as a beverage but is available in extract form. Therapeutic doses are traditionally believed to be reached by drinking 1 teaspoon of green tea leaf in 1-cup boiling water 5 times or more daily.

Tea Tree Oil

Botanical Name:
Melaleuca alternifolia

Properties:
Analgesic, Antibacterial, Antifungal, Anti-inflammatory, Antimicrobial, Antiseptic, Antiviral, Expectorant, Immunostimulant, Insecticide, Vulnerary

Traditional Use:
Tea tree oil is traditionally used in aromatherapy to reduce air borne infectious agents.

Tea Tree has been blended at a rate of 5% oil, 5% peroxide, to 90% base to create a traditional topical treatment for infections.

Crushed Tea Tree leaves have traditionally been used as a snuff like inhalant to reduce the duration of respiratory infections like the common cold, influenza, and pneumonia.

Tea tree oil is traditionally used as a broad-spectrum antimicrobial against a wide variety of bacterial, fungus, and viruses. It is traditionally included in salves and ointments, and natural cleaning products.

Tea Tree oil has been used as a traditional topical ointment or lotion component to treat outbreaks of herpes acting to minimize the number and duration of flares.

In addition to its own infection fighting properties, Tea Tree leaves are used as a traditional infusion to stimulate the body's own immune system.

Tea Tree oil is traditionally used in vapor therapy to ease congestion and speed healing in congestive infections like bronchitis, colds, and influenza.

Part Used:
Branch Tips, Leaf - Oil

Side Effects:
Tea Tree Oil is for external use only.

Tea Tree Oil is not recommended for use by women who are pregnant or nursing.

Tea Tree Oil may not be recommended for use in topical preparations for young children.

Tea Tree Oil should is not recommended for use on deep wounds.

Tea Tree oil should not be used near the eyes, ears, or nose.

Tea Tree Oil can cause skin burning, dryness, irritation, itching, redness, or stinging in some people.

Ingestion of Tea Tree Oil may cause diarrhea, coma, and death.

Additional uses and side effects may exist but further research is necessary to determine the exact properties and effects of use.

General:
Tea Tree oil comes from the leaves of an evergreen shrub commonly called Tea Tree. It is native Asia and Australia but cultivated in other regions. Hardy to zone 9, it is not particular regarding soil composition but does prefer good drainage, consistent moisture, and full sun. It can be propagated by seed sown indoors in the fall or by cuttings taken in the mid summer that contain a heel of the previous year's growth.

Tea Tree has been used for centuries by the aborigines as a topical treatment and traditional supplement. Tea Tree oil is extracted from the leaves by steam distillation and is used topically and in cleaning products.

Thyme, French Thyme, Garden Thyme, Red Thyme, Rubbed Thyme, Spanish Thyme, Tomillo, Van Ajwayan, White Thyme

Botanical Name:
Thymus vulgaris

Properties:
Analgesic, Antibacterial, Antifungal, Antioxidant, Antiperspirant, Antiseptic, Antispasmodic, Antitussive, Antiviral, Aphrodisiac, Cancer, Carminative, Depurative, Diaphoretic, Digestive, Emmenagogue, Expectorant, Hypertensive, Insect Repellant, Nervine, Sedative, Vermifuge

Traditional Use:
Thyme contains compounds that are used to help dilate the bronchial passages, sooth respiratory ailments, fight infection, expel excess mucus, and suppress nighttime coughs in commercial and traditional syrups for conditions like asthma, bronchitis, colds, congestion, and influenza.

Thyme oil inhalants are traditionally used to help shorten the duration and severity of common infections like colds and influenza.

Thyme is often used as part of a household cleaner disinfectant recipe.

Thyme has been used in traditional air purification and disinfectant treatments.

Thyme oil inhalants are traditionally used to help shorten the duration and severity of common infections like colds and influenza.

Part Used:
Flower, Leaf, Stem

Side Effects:
Thyme is not recommended for use by women who are pregnant or nursing.

Thyme can cause an allergic reaction in some people.

Thyme oil may elevate the blood pressure.

Overuse of thyme can effect the menstrual cycles in some women

The oils isolated from the Thyme plant can be toxic and should not be ingested but the herb itself is generally considered safe.

Additional uses and side effects may exist but further research is necessary to determine the exact properties and effects of use.

General:
Thyme is native to the Mediterranean but is cultivated in many areas of the world. Hardy to zone 7, it is grown in containers in cooler regions. It prefers sandy or loamy soil, good drainage, and full sun. It can be propagated by seed, spring division, cuttings in the mid summer that contain a heel of the last years growth or by layering at any time during the growing season.

Thyme is harvested as a culinary seasoning and as a liquid extract for use in traditional supplements. The oils are used in perfumery or in traditional topical preparations. The leaves and flowers are eaten as a raw vegetable or added to recipes as a flavoring.

The oils are extracted through steam distillation for use in aromatherapy. Red Thyme and White Thyme oil come from the same plant. The alteration in coloring is due to oxidation during the extraction and methods used when processing of the oils. Red Thyme oil contains stronger antiseptic properties and is traditionally used for disinfection. White Thyme oil has more of the impurities removed and tends to have a milder action making it preferred in many traditional treatments.

Tribulus, Bindii, Bullhead, Caltrop, Cat's Head, Devil's Eyelashes, Devil's Thorn, Devil's Weed, Gouthead, Puncturevine, Puncture Weed

Botanical Name:
Tribulus terrestris

Properties:
Abortifacient, Androgen Production, Antibacterial, Antiviral, Aphrodisiac, Astringent, Cardiac, Carminative, Demulcent, Diuretic, Estrogenic, Galactogogue, Hypotensive, Steroidal Saponins, Stimulant

Traditional Use:
Tribulus has been shown to have antibacterial and antiviral properties that make it a traditional tea for use in treating internal and external bacterial and viral infections.

Part Used:
Fruit, Leaf, Seed

Side Effects:
Tribulus is not recommended for use by women who are pregnant or nursing.

Tribulus seed has been used as an abortifacient in some cultures.

Tribulus is not recommended for use by people who are taking nitroglycerine or have a heart condition.

Tribulus may act on the hormones and is not recommended for use by men who have prostate problems.

Tribulus may affect blood sugar levels.

The fruit of the Tribulus is not for internal use.

Additional uses and side effects may exist but further research is necessary to determine the exact properties and effects of use.

General:
Tribulus is native to Europe and has been naturalized to other parts of the world where it is considered an invasive weed by some. It is not particular regarding soil composition but does prefer full sun and consistent moisture. Tribulus can be propagated by seeds and will self sow readily if given its own place in the garden.

Tribulus leaves and shoots are eaten as a cooked vegetable and the seeds are ground into flour. The whole plant is harvested, dried, and powdered for use as a traditional supplement.

Usnea, Beard Moss, Old Man's Beard, Tree Moss, Tree's Dandruff, Usnia, Women's Long Hair

Botanical Name:
Usnea barbata

Properties:
Analgesic, Antibacterial, Antibiotic, Antifungal, Anti-inflammatory, Antiviral, Expectorant, Febrifuge

Traditional Uses:
Usnea has traditionally been used to provide general pain relief and helps to alleviate congestion in conditions like asthma, bronchitis, colds, and influenza. Usnea also has antibacterial and antiviral properties that make it a traditional supplement to shorten the length of common infections including bronchitis, colds, influenza, and pneumonia.

Parts Used:
Whole

Side Effects:
Usnea is not recommended for use by women who are pregnant or nursing.

Usnea may cause abdominal pain, nausea, fatigue, muscle weakness, and liver damage.

Additional uses and side effects may exist but further research is necessary to determine the exact properties and effects of use.

General:
Usnea is a type of algae and fungus combination that grow together on trees and are often termed lichen. The whole plant is used in traditional supplements and is most frequently used as an alcohol extract.

Wild Garlic

Common Names:
Ramsons, Wild Garlic

Botanical Name:
Allium ursinum

Properties:
Antibacterial, Antifungal, Antimicrobial, Antioxidant, Antiseptic, Antiviral, Antiseptic, Antispasmodic, Astringent, Cholagogue, Cholesterol, Depurative, Diaphoretic, Diuretic, Emmenagogue, Expectorant, Febrifuge, Hypotensive, Immunostimulant, Insect Repellant, Rubefacient, Stimulant, Vermifuge

Traditional Uses:
Wild Garlic contains a broad spectrum antimicrobial and has been used in traditional supplements to shorten the length of infections.

The juices of the Wild Garlic have been used as disinfecting agent in household cleansing products.

Wild Garlic has traditionally been used in dietary plans to boost the body's immune response helping to ward off common infections.

Parts Used:
Bulb, Whole

Side Effects:
Wild Garlic is not recommended for use beyond dietary by women who are pregnant or nursing. Wild Garlic is a known uterus stimulant.

Wild Garlic is not recommended for use beyond dietary in children's treatments.

Overuse of Wild Garlic may cause heartburn in some people.

Overuse of Wild Garlic may burn the skin in some people.

Garlic may cause bad breath, body odor, upset stomach, and rarely allergic reactions in some people.

Wild Garlic may reduce the blood clotting ability. Do not use garlic supplements if you are planning to have surgery, dental work, or have a bleeding disorder.

Additional uses and side effects may exist but further research is necessary to determine the exact properties and effects of use.

General:
Wild Garlic is a bulb plant native to Western Asia and Europe but cultivated elsewhere for its ability to deliver higher potency than commonly cultivated garlic with less aroma. Hardy to zone 5, Wild Garlic is not particular regarding sun conditions but does prefer sandy or loamy soil and consistent moisture. It can be propagated by seed or by bulb division.

The juices of the Wild Garlic have been used as an insect repellant primarily against insects like moths. The bulbs, leaves, and flowers are eaten as a raw or cooked vegetable though the aroma increases as the plant ripens.

Wild Garlic is similar in composition and uses to cultivated Garlic but has a milder aroma and weaker action making it more common for use in traditional treatments given over a longer period.

Woad, Ben Lan Gen, Chinese Indigo, Dyer's Woad, Farberwaid, Glastum, Hierba Pastel, Indigo Woad, Isatis, Quing Dai

Botanical Name:
Isatis tinctoria

Properties:
Analgesic, Antibacterial, Antibiotic, Anti-inflammatory, Antiviral, Cancer, Colorant, Febrifuge, Immunostimulant

Traditional Use:
Woad is believed to stimulate the immune system and act as an antiviral in traditional treatments for colds, influenza, and other viral infections.

Woad is traditionally used as a short-term antibiotic to treat a wide range of infections including bacterial and viral infections.

Part Used:
Leaf, Root

Side Effects:
Woad is not recommended for use by women who are pregnant or nursing.

Woad is not recommended for use in children's treatments.

Woad contains aspirin like substances and is not recommended for use by people with an allergy to aspirin.

Woad is not recommended for people on blood thinning medication.

Additional uses and side effects may exist but further research is necessary to determine the exact properties and effects of use.

General:
Woad is native to Asia but is naturalized to Europe and North America where it has been cultivated as a blue dye product for thousands of years.

The leaf and root are harvested for use fresh or dried in traditional supplements. Alcohol extracts are undergoing study as a potential treatment for slowing the growth of cancer cells.

Wormwood – Sweet, Absinthe, Ajenjo, Annual Mugwort, Annual Wormwood, Artemisia, Chinese Wormwood, Huang Hua Guo, Quing Hao, Sweet Annie, Sweet Wormwood

Botanical Name:
Artemisia annua

Properties:
Antibacterial, Antibiotic, Antifungal, Antiparasitic, Antiviral, Sedative, Vermifuge

Traditional Uses:
Sweet Wormwood is traditionally used in topical and supplement preparations to treat bacterial, fungal, parasitic, and viral infections.

Parts Used:
Leaf, Flower, Stem

Side Effects:
Sweet Wormwood is not recommended for use by women who are pregnant or nursing.

Sweet Wormwood may cause an allergic reaction in some people.

Additional uses and side effects may exist but further research is necessary to determine the exact properties and effects of use.

General:
Sweet Wormwood is native to Asia but has naturalized throughout much of the world. The flower, leaf, and stem are used in traditional treatments.

Using Natural Ingredients

The barks, flowers, leaves and roots that have been used for centuries as traditional supplements are still easily obtainable from health food stores, organic growers, and even in the wild. Many of plants used in traditional supplements are also easy to grow. Whether you have a windowsill garden or acreage waiting to be farmed, you can selectively grow, harvest, and process many of the traditional supplements successfully used for thousands of years to treat common ailments.

There are numerous ways of using plant products as supplements. You can use plant products as a drink, flavoring, culinary seasoning, aromatherapy treatment, and so forth. Nearly any supplement preparation you purchase at the store can be made from scratch using fresh plant products from sources you know you can trust to grow them without the addition of harmful chemical treatments. There are numerous natural product recipe guides available, including my Green & Natural book series that include simple recipes you can create to replace almost every supplement that you use.

The first step in making natural supplements is to know the type of supplements you need. The second step is to obtain the plant parts that you will use in the creation of the supplements. Most people quickly decide they want to create their own supplements starting at the beginning. That means growing their own plants to harvest, process, and use.

Each type of flower, herb, shrub, or tree will need a slightly different environment and handling for optimal growth. Propagation of plants is another entire subject that cannot be completely addressed here. If you are interested in propagating many types of plants using different methods, you should obtain a guide to help you along the way. Seed propagation is among the most common and cost effective ways to get a garden started so we will illustrate how easily you can cultivate your own supplement garden from seeds.

To create the perfect supplement garden for your needs, you must decide what plants you want to include. The compendium provides details about plants that have traditionally been used as supplements to address common conditions. You should compile a list of your preferred plants from the pages of the compendium.

As a starting organic grower, you will want to narrow the list to include those plants that fit within your climate and the space that you have available for growing.

You will want to consider the growth patterns of the plants you select for your supplement garden. Planning the types of plants included in the garden helps to ensure you have an adequate harvest during each season and do not need to replace exhausted plants. The two most common classifications of plants you will encounter are the annual and the perennial.

Some plants are annual plants. An annual plant is one that completes its entire life cycle in one year and then dies. Annuals usually grow quickly. When growing annuals for supplement use, you can harvest the entire plant each season. You will start the next season with a new plant. You can even harvest the seeds and process them yourself for next year.

If you live in a warmer climate, you should remember that a plant that is considered an annual in most regions might actually be a perennial in your area. You will want to confirm how the particular plants you select grow in your region before completely harvesting it in case the plant might yield more growth.

A perennial plant is a plant that continues to grow year after year. Many of the plants in the compendium are perennial plants. In some regions, perennial plants will simply continue to grow, going through slower and faster cycles of growth depending on the season. In other regions, perennial plants may enter a period of dormancy followed by a period of new growth. You will usually not want to harvest all of the parts of a perennial plant. You should take only as much as you need from the plant and leave the rest so the plant can continue to grow, regularly producing new crops for you to use.

Once you have a compiled a listing of the plants that you want to cultivate, you can obtain seedlings from a grower or purchase seeds from a reputable supplier. Most home supplement growers prefer to grow their plants from seeds.

The cost of growing a plant from seed is often much lower than the cost of purchasing seedlings or adult plants. In addition, when you grow a plant yourself, you know the exact history of the plant. You can feel confident that no chemicals were used during the growing process and that the plant you will be using as a supplement is healthy.

If you are growing from seed, you will need to gather a few items.

Seeds
Potting Medium
Coverage
Light Source

You will want to obtain containers that are safe for plant growth. There are many available growing containers. All natural, biodegradable plant starters are among the most environmentally friendly and chemical free options. These tend to be more costly than some other options and may not be worthwhile if you are keeping the mature plants indoors instead of transferring them to an outside space. There is a wide variety of seeding options available and you should select the one that will be most useful in your garden plan. The biggest consideration when selecting containers for supplement growing is to ensure that they are not made of a plastic product that can degrade and cause damage to your plants or cause the plant to ingest chemicals that will then contaminate any products you make from that plant.

The container you select should allow for water drainage. Commercially sold planting cups are usually created with a drainage feature. If you are making your own planting cups, you will want to put a few small holes in the bottom to allow excess water to drain away from the roots.

You will need to purchase pre-mixed seeding medium or harvest your own from a nutrient rich area of your yard. If you are a regular gardener, you know where the best potting soil can be found. If you are a beginner, purchasing pre-mixed organic seed starter is typically a better choice. Seeding mix should be light enough to allow for good air circulation but not so light that it creates an unsustainable rooting medium for the plants as they grow.

Fill each of your seed cups ¾ of the way full with seeding mix. Gently tap or press the soil to ensure there are no air pockets. Air pockets can cause the seed to drop too deeply into the soil and may make it difficult for young roots to find sufficient nutrients. A young root that encounters an air pocket is likely to wither and die weakening the plant.

Most seeds do best if you soak them in water for a few hours before planting. You may want to soak my seeds and filled soil cups at the same time. Make certain all of the products you will be using are well saturated with clean water.

The water that you use should be as free of chemicals as possible. If you have access to a clean stream or spring, this is an excellent place to obtain planting water. You could also collect rainwater to use in your garden. If necessary, most stores sell natural spring water.

After your seeds and soil are well moistened, you will sow the seeds. Most seeds do well with just a light covering of potting medium. A standard guide is to place the seed 3 times deeper than the size of the seed. Very tiny seeds are just barely placed into the soil while larger seeds are as much as ¼ inch into the medium.

Your seeds will need moisture protection during the early stages of development. You can purchase pre-made mini greenhouses or make a plastic tent to protect the seeds during germination and early development.

The seeds are now ready to do their job. You should place them in a warm area where they will not be disturbed. Seeds germinate at different rates so you will want to check on the seedlings often. A germinating seed requires warmth and moisture but does not need large amounts of light. Once the seedling emerges, it will require much more light.

If you are lucky enough to have a sunny area, natural light works well for most seedlings. Most indoor locations do not receive an adequate amount of light for new seedlings. You can use growing bulbs to provide light supplementation during the first weeks of seedling development. Each seedling will have varying light needs and you will want to check the exact growth requirements of the plants you have selected for your supplement garden.

A simple way to determine if your seedlings are getting enough light is to watch how they grow. Plants that are not receiving sufficient light will begin to become leggy as they search for a light source. That means they will grow tall, weak stems in an attempt to capture more light. If you notice your plants are growing tall but not thickening, chances are good that they are not receiving adequate light and you will need to add supplemental lighting.

Over the first few weeks, you will want to make sure that your seedlings stay moist but not saturated. The easiest way to keep the seedlings moist but not saturated is through bottom watering. If you have not already placed your growing cups on a tray, you will want to do so now.

The tray should have edges about as high as a cookie sheet. Pour water into the tray around the potting cups. This allows the soil to absorb the water the plant needs through the drainage holes in a cup or through the cup itself if you are using biodegradable planting cups. Watering from the top increases the likelihood of washing the seeds too deeply into the soil or damaging the newly emerged plants.

Each morning and afternoon, check the water level in the seedling tray. If too much water remains in the bottom of the pan, you will need to lessen the amount you give at each watering. If the pan becomes dry too quickly, you will either need to give more water at each watering or water more frequently. The goal is to provide enough moisture to keep the soil damp but not soggy.

If you live in a very moist climate, you may want to remove the germinating plastic once the seedlings emerge. If you live in a dry climate, are propagating during a cold month, or are growing delicate plants, you may want to leave the germinating plastic on the plants until they have developed their second set of leaves. By the time the second set of leaves has developed, the root system is typically strong enough to support the plant. If you do choose to leave the moisture retaining cover on the plants, you will need to create vents to ensure that your seedlings and potting medium are not too wet.

Once the second set of leaves have developed on your seedling it is time to begin "hardening" the plant. If you are planning to transplant the seedling outdoors, hardening is a critical step. If you are planning to maintain an indoor garden, hardening is still important but not critical to the success of your seedling.

Hardening means giving your seedlings the opportunity to become strong enough to survive natural environmental changes. A nice first step to begin hardening your plants is to open a nearby window or allow a fan to blow close to but not directly at the plants. This gives the plants to chance to adapt to changes in airflow and temperature.

If the seedlings are going to be indoor plants, you can gradually increase the number of hours that they are exposed to the airflow.

If you will be transplanting the seedlings to an outdoor garden, you will need to adapt them to the outside conditions. Once they seem to be bearing up well to indirect air and alterations in temperature, you should take seedlings outdoors for a few hours at a time. Spend a week or two gradually increasing the amount of time the plants stay outdoors. Once they are spending most of the day outside and any chance of extremely cold temperatures or severe storms have passed, you can transplant the seedlings to their permanent home.

Select the strongest seedlings to transplant. Some people pull out the hardier seedlings for transplanting and give the less hardy seedlings a bit more time to strengthen while others simply discard the weaker seedlings. Both methods have their positive points so you should do what works best for your ultimate growing plans.

Before you plant your seedling, you will want to pinch off the lowest set or sets of leaves. These nodes will grow roots once the plant is placed in the deeper soil of the permanent planting location.

You will pre-dig the holes for your seedlings whether you are planting them indoors or out. The hole should be deep enough to cover the bottom nodes you exposed when pinched the lower leaves. This deep planting will create a stronger plant and compensate for any legginess the plants developed reaching for light as seedlings.

You will want to ensure that the transplant soil is free of chemicals, weeds, and other contaminants. You will also want to use the best potting soil for your seedlings. A good mixture is 1 part vermiculate, 1 part perlite and 1 part potting mix.

If you have planted the seedlings in biodegradable grow cups, you will likely pull out all of the weaker plants and place the grow cup in your prepared location.

If you have planted the seedlings in a home made grow cup, you will need to turn the cup to release the seedling for transplant. You should use care to not to tug on the stems or leaves when removing the plant from the cup. Pulling on the plant during transplant will harm the delicate structures that the plant needs to survive. You might need to use a knife or spoon to help release the plant and lever it out of the cup.

You might notice the roots of the seedling are tightly bound in the shape of the planting cup. If the roots are tightly bound, you may want to loosen them before placing the plant into its permanent location. You can take your finger and gently tug the roots loose the same way you would untangle long hair. You can also take a clean pair of gardening scissors and make a straight cut on the four sides of the root ball by beginning at the bottom and working toward your seedling. This process helps to agitate the roots and encourages new growth. It also helps to spread the roots so that they grow outward from the plant, penetrating the soil in every direction. Penetration in all directions helps to give your plant the highest potential for gathering nutrients and water from the surrounding soil.

After you have worked the roots, place the selected seedling into the prepared hole and backfill with the potting mixture you have selected. You will want to pat the soil around the plant to remove any air pockets. You may want to mulch around outdoor plants to help them retain moisture and discourage weed growth.

Water the soil around the plants at least once a day for the first couple of weeks. The amount of water necessary will vary depending on the location, climate, type of plant, and soil conditions. The plants should stay moist but not soggy during the first weeks outdoors. Watering the soil instead of the plant helps prevent damage to the seedling. Think of it as a method similar to the bottom watering you completed on your newly emerged seedlings.

Harvesting & Drying Herbs

One of the biggest questions about homegrown plants is when to harvest. Many plants can be harvested at the beginning of the flowering season, though some are better in the middle or end of the season. Each entry gives a general idea on appropriate harvest times for a particular plant.

In general, if you are harvesting for the leaves or buds, you should harvest the plant before it blooms. If you are harvesting for the flowers & petals, you should harvest the plant in the middle of the growing season. If you are seeking seeds or roots, harvest them after the blooms have died off.

If you observe your plants, you should be able to begin to recognize the peak time for harvesting. Like a ripe tomato, all plant parts have a point where they are perfect for harvesting. This peak point is when the beneficial compounds are at the highest concentration.

The time of day you harvest can change the success of the supplement you are making. Some plants are at their richest early in the morning while others become richer as the warmth and moisture of the day give them the strength they need.

You will want to observe the specific type of plant you are harvesting to determine what time of day might be the peak time for that plant. The default time to harvest when you are not sure is mid-morning. This is the time after the dew has evaporated but before the plants begin to wilt from the heat of the day.

You will decide how to harvest based on the type of plant, method of drying you plan, and ultimate use of the plants.

If you are primarily interested in only the flowers & leaves of the plant, you can pluck these off the mother plant and allow the remainder to continue growing in the hopes of getting another harvest later in the season. If the plant is an annual or you need the roots, you will harvest the whole plant. If the plant is a perennial, you should use care not to over harvest since this increases the risk of killing the plant.

Once you have harvested the plant parts you will use, you should clean them. If you have purchased plants from another grower, you will want to make certain any chemicals used during the growing process are cleaned off your plant parts. Even if you grow the plants yourself, you will want to wash the plants to remove any bugs, eggs, soil, and other contaminants that might have gotten in with your plants.

You can pat the plants dry with a clean, soft cloth or simply shake the excess water off the plant and allow them to finish drip-drying while you prepare whatever next step you will take with your plants.

One of the most common methods of using plants as supplements is as a dried product that will be made into teas, infusions, decoctions, or other products. The purpose of drying your plant products is to remove the fluids, preserve the beneficial compounds and extend the useful life of the plant parts.

There is some confusion related to using fresh or dried plant parts when making products like extracts, oil infusions, and other supplements. All fresh plant products will contain some amount of water. The type of plant part you are using will dictate how much of the part is fluid and how much is plant. The presence of water will dilute the potency when you make supplements like an extract or tincture. You can use fresh plant parts but most people find they attain a higher efficiency and need less storage room when they dry the plant matter before processing it into various supplements.

There are many ways to dry plant parts. Each of them has benefits and drawbacks. The three basic methods that are most often used for drying plants are air-drying, speed drying, and hang drying.

Air Drying Plants

Air-drying is exactly how it sounds. You will expose the parts of the plant to the air to allow the moisture to evaporate. A few plants do well when air and sun are combined during the process but most should be kept out of direct sunlight since it can evaporate or damage the beneficial compounds you are trying to obtain.

Air-drying is the slowest method of drying plant products but it often allows the plant parts to retain more beneficial compounds.

Before starting the air-drying process, you should decide where you are going to dry the plants. If the weather is just right, you may be able to dry the plants outside away from direct sunlight and the elements. More often, you will want to select an area inside the home where the plant will not be disturbed during drying.

The biggest consideration is that the area you select must be very dry. Plants will not dry properly in a space with high humidity.

The second consideration is that the area should not get extreme air movement from nature, fans, door closures, people, or another source. As the plant parts dry, they will become light. A good breeze will scatter the plants and ruin the project.

You should also consider the container you will use to dry your plants. There are many different types of air-drying racks available for purchase. Many of these allow you to stack the plants for drying. These are very convenient and some are even pretty. Depending on the amount of air-drying you will do, purchasing drying racks can become costly. If you want to keep costs low or will only be drying plants occasionally, you can make your own drying bins. A simple rack can be made by layering a clean cotton towel or waxed paper inside a shallow cookie sheet or even a cardboard box. Whatever bins you choose must not be able to absorb the compounds from your plant, must not contaminate the plant, must allow you to dry the plant parts in one layer not a pile, and must be durable enough to withstand the turning or agitation of the plant parts.

Once you have selected the container for your drying processes, you will need to finish preparing the plant parts.

The cleaned, dried herbs will need to be broken down into smaller pieces. It is often beneficial to break the plants into smaller pieces prior to drying. This not only saves you time later, it speeds the drying process since smaller parts give more air exposure and thus a faster drying process. You can pull the leaves, flowers, and stems apart with your hands or use a pair of clean shears to achieve the right size.

Place the plant pieces into the prepared container in one thin layer. This helps ensure more plant parts are exposed to the air. The more parts exposed to the air, the faster the plant materials will dry. The faster the plant materials dry, the less likely they are to develop mold growth.

Different plants will dry at different rates. You will want to agitate or turn your plant parts at least one time each day. The more moisture you have in the air or in the plant, the more frequently you will want to turn the mixture. The goal with agitating the plant parts is to ensure that everything dries evenly and quickly.

It is important that the plants dry as quickly as possible. If you enter a very humid period during the drying process, you may need to place the drying containers in the oven to help prevent excess moisture build up and mold growth.

Oven Assisted Plant Drying
You can speed dry the plant parts in the oven. This is not one of my favorite methods because you run the risk of cooking the plant parts instead of simply drying them. There are times when oven drying may be the only logical solution like when a high humidity day hits in the middle of the drying process. It may be a better choice to risk cooking the herbs rather than risk losing the entire batch to mold.

If you choose to use the oven assist drying method, you need to make certain your oven is clean and free of chemicals. Any chemicals in the oven may pollute your plant products.

You should turn the oven on to its lowest setting and leave the door open to its first 'notch' or about 4 inches. This helps to allow air into the drying process and to keep the oven from becoming too warm.

You will need to array your plant parts as thinly as possible on the drying mat. A perforated oven-safe tray works best for oven assist drying. If you do not have an oven-safe tray, you can layer clean cotton or paper towels across the oven racks. Place the plant products onto the chosen holder.

The herbs will dry very quickly in the oven so you should check them every couple of minutes to ensure they do not over dry or 'cook'. The amount of time you will need to dry the plants will depend on the type of plant product you are using, the amount of moisture remaining in the plants, the humidity in the air, and other factors.

When you check the plants you will want to agitate them like you would during air-drying. This will help the plant parts to dry more evenly. If you are using a soft cloth and can safely pick up the drying tray, just bouncing the plant parts a few times may be a sufficient method of agitation. If you are using a solid rack, turn the herbs every few minutes.

Speed Drying Herbs
Food dehydrators have completely changed the way some people dry their herbs. A dehydrator follows the same basic concept as air-drying it just does the job much more quickly. The dehydrator forces warm, dry air around the plant parts. This helps to remove the moisture from the plants more quickly and actually makes a more pleasing final product for some plant parts like oily fruit rinds, wood bark, and nuts.

The dehydrator must have a fan and allow you to set the heat setting extremely low or else you will cook your plants just as you would in an overheated oven. If the dehydrator you are using has a recommendation in the manual for drying herbs, you should start with those instructions and then adapt the settings to suit your particular needs. If there are no recommendations, start the process with the temperature on the lowest setting, usually around 90°, and gradually increase the temperature if you feel the plants are drying too slowly.

You will spread the plant parts onto the dehydrator trays in a single layer. You should make your layer loose so there is plenty of room for airflow to reach all sides of the plants.

The dehydrator will complete the drying process much more quickly than air-drying. You should check the plants every 15 – 20 minutes. At each check, you may want to rotate the trays. The plant parts closest to the heat source will dry more quickly and rotating the trays helps to distribute the airflow & heat. You should remove the plant parts as they become dry enough for use.

Hang Drying Plants
Hang Drying is an easy way to dry plants that works well if you have plenty of space and a controlled room where you can hang the plants. Hang drying also helps to produce a stronger final product when you are going to be using only the flowers & leaves.

You will want to be certain there are no contaminants in the room for the plants to absorb during drying and that the air is very low in humidity. I use hang drying in the winter months since heating the house often serves a dual purpose of removing humidity from the air. Drying herbs in a closed house also helps to brighten and freshen the house naturally.

When you harvest for hang drying, you will leave longer stems on the plants. The stems will be used for the hanging. Cut each plant as close to the same length as you can.

Gather the ends of the stems together. You can use a pasta measure to judge how much you have gathered clumping about 1 serving worth per hanging group. If you make the hanging group too large, it will take longer to dry and you risk ruining the batch if the air cannot reach the middle plants.

Tie the gathered stems into a bouquet about 2 inches from the ends using natural string or jute. You will want to tie the stems tightly enough that they do not fall out of the clump but not so tightly that you break the stem. Leave an extra length of string to hook the clump to your hanger.

The stems will shrink as they dry so you may want to check the bundle occasionally to ensure that the tie has not loosened so much that you are losing stems.

Hang the herbs upside down with the cut stems facing toward the ceiling. This helps the compounds in the plant travel toward the leaves & flowers strengthening the final product.

Hang drying makes seed capture easy if you plan to propagate a new batch of plants. Place a bin, paper bag, or cardboard box underneath the hanging plant. The bin will capture any plant parts or seeds that fall off when the plant becomes dry enough to release them.

The amount of time necessary for hang drying will depend on the temperature of the area, humidity in the air, moisture in the plant, density of the plant, and other factors. You should check the plants regularly to see if they are ready for storage.

Storing Dried Herbs

Each plant product will dry at a different rate and you should check often to see if any of the matter is ready for use or storage. You will become adept at judging the progress of the drying by sight. You should be able to see & feel a gradual reduction in the moisture of the plant parts.

Select a leaf or flower and hold it between your thumb and forefinger. Gently rub your fingers back and forth. The leaf or flower will break into tiny pieces without much effort. It should not powder. If the plant parts powder as soon as you touch them, they are too dry. Over-drying the plant parts diminishes the power of the active compounds.

At times, you will be drying flower buds or berries. These will appear different when dry from a leaf or flower petal. Select a berry or flower bud and look at it closely. It should look and feel like a hardened raisin. When it feels like a hardened raisin, it is ready for storage or use.

Stems and twigs dry differently than other plant parts. Select a stem or twig that appears to be dry and try to snap it into smaller pieces. Fully dried stems & twigs will snap easily much like a piece of uncooked spaghetti.

Seeds and nuts can be dried and broken to check their readiness for storage. Select a nut or seed and place it on a hard surface like a cutting board and then attempt to crush it with a kitchen mallet, the bottom of a ceramic cup, or the side of your shears. Nuts & seeds should break into a powder that does not clump easily. If the powder is still clumping, there are likely too many oils in the nut or seed and you should allow them to dry further before storage. If the powder is fine and easily sifted, the seeds or nuts are ready to be ground into flour for storage or use or stored whole until you are ready for them.

If you are still not certain your plant parts are ready for storage, you can select a small amount of the plant and place it in a clean, dry glass jar. Seal the lid tightly and place the jar in a warm, sunny location. If moisture condenses inside the jar over the first few hours, the plant is not ready for storage. If no moisture appears, the plant part is dry enough for storage.

You should store your newly dried plant product in a way that will not allow moisture or contaminants to permeate back into the dried goods. Some people use special stainless steel storage cans while others make "bags" from waxed paper. Porcelain, ceramic, and glass are other common choices. You should choose whatever storage method works best in your household. You do need to select a storage container that blocks moisture, light, and chemical contaminants.

Most correctly dried pant parts will retain many of their beneficial compounds for 1 year after the harvesting and storage date.

Freezing Plants

Sometimes, plant parts need to be harvested at a time that is not conducive to drying or the parts just do not dry properly. When this happens, another option is to freeze the plants.

Some people make freezing their primary method of storage for all of their harvests. If you do not have a dry room, live in a moist climate, or are unable to air dry the plant parts for another reason, freezing may be an alternative for you. You should remember that freezing is not technically a drying method and a great deal of the moisture will remain in the plant parts making any supplement made from freeze-dried plants weaker than their traditionally dried counterparts do.

Freezing is actually a simpler method of storing. You will harvest and clean the plant parts the same way that you do in any storage process. After the excess water has been removed, strip the leaves, petals, and any other plant parts you plan to save. Place the usable pieces in the freezer storage container you have selected. The faster you freeze the parts the better, so a deep freezer or the quick freeze shelf in some side-by-side freezers is a good choice. The plant parts should be good for use for 3-4 months.

Delivery Mediums

Herbal Tea & Infusions

Once you have dried your plant parts, you will want to decide how to use them. Teas and infusions are two of the most common methods of using dried supplements. Making a natural tea or infusion allows you to obtain the benefits of the plant compounds while enjoying a variety of flavor sensations.

Infusions are not just for ingesting. You can use an infusion in the bath, in creams or lotions, as a wash, for cleaning, or for almost any other activity that can benefit from the compounds contained in the plants and can support a liquid medium.

An infusion is made using the soft plant parts. These are parts like the flower or leaf.

You will need to decide the source of the water you will use to make your tea or infusion. Filtered water, spring water, and rainwater are all good choices. The primary concern with water is to ensure it has as few contaminates as possible.

You will want to choose a teapot or kettle for heating water that is not going to degrade and release chemicals into the final product. Glass, stainless steel, and ceramic are all common choices.

Warm the water to boiling in the kettle and then remove it from the heat.

You will want to get a tea ball to contain your plant parts or tea strainer to help you remove the plant parts from the finished drink.

Tea balls tend to keep the plant parts together and leave far fewer 'clumps' in the finished drink but they also tend to compress the plant parts and make releasing the beneficial compounds more difficult.

Tea strainers allow the plant parts to move freely in the water, releasing more of their compounds but also tend to allow small plant parts to escape into the finished drink.

Either option works well and the one you choose will be based on your personal preference and needs.

You will choose the plant or combination of plants that provide the benefits you want from a supplement. These will vary greatly between people. You can even add a base tea just for the flavor! Regardless of the type of plants you are using, you will need between ¾ and 1 teaspoon of dried plant product per cup of liquid.

If you have not crumbled the plant parts before, you will want to break them into smaller pieces now. Smaller pieces gives the water more access to the plant parts and helps the compounds to release more easily.

You can add the dried pieces directly to your kettle as long as it has been removed from the heat source or place them in a cup and pour the water from the kettle on top.

Placing the herbs into the kettle, whether loose or in the tea ball, helps to prevent the oils from evaporating during steeping but also leaves residue inside the kettle that may interfere with the next supplement you make if you do not clean the kettle well after each use.

Pouring the water over the leaves in the cup allows more of the beneficial compounds to escape into the air but helps to prevent cross contamination between supplement usages since cups will usually be easier to wash than a kettle.

Either method of getting plant parts into contact with the water works and you should choose the option that suits you the best.

Allow the leaves to steep in the water for between 5 minutes and 6 hours depending on the supplement you are trying to create. A traditional tea is not as strong as an infusion and often an ingested supplement will be weaker than a topical preparation.

Once your drink is steeped to your desired strength, remove the plant parts from the liquid, flavor to taste, and enjoy.

Cold Infusion

Many plants release their compounds best to warm water. Occasionally you may want to use a plant that does not release as well to heat. Some plants that are high in mucilage content or bitter compounds seem to do better when the compounds are infused in cold fluid. These are often referenced as digestive in descriptions.

A cold infusion is made by soaking the selected plant parts in room temperature or cooler liquid instead of hot water. You do not need to limit yourself to water. Some cold infusions are made with milk, juices, or another preferred liquid.

You will use the same proportions of plant parts and liquid as you do for a hot infusion. You will prepare the plant parts following the same processes. You will even consume the cold infusion the same way you do a hot infusion. The two major differences when making a cold infusion are that you will use cold water, milk, or another liquid instead of hot and you will allow the plant parts to steep for a longer period than you do with a warm infusion.

Decoction

A decoction is made with plant parts that are simmered in water. A decoction is usually used to extract the compounds from tougher plant parts like barks, roots, seeds, and wood. These plant parts are tougher than leaves or flowers and tend to require more heat to release the beneficial compounds.

The amount of plant product to water will vary depending on the plant you are using and the desired results. An average is 3 teaspoons of dried plant pieces for each 1 cup of water. You will want to adjust this ratio to suit the plant parts you are using and the results you need.

Tougher plant parts should be chopped finer when you begin. It is common to grate or powder decoction components before adding them to the water.

When making a decoction, you will simmer the plant parts instead of adding the plants to the water once it is already hot. This helps to force the tougher plants to release their compounds.

Add the plant parts and water to your simmering pot. A glass, stainless steel, or ceramic pot works well. You should place a lid on the pot to help prevent more loss of active compounds than necessary.

Simmer the decoction, keeping the heat just below a boil. The amount of time you will simmer the plant parts depends on a variety of factors including the plant's toughness and the strength you want from the finished product. Your goal is to reduce the fluids in the mixture. A traditional decoction is complete when the water has been reduced by ½. In other words, if you start with 1 cup of water, you will finish with ½ cup.

Strain the plant parts from the fluid as soon as you remove the mixture from the heat. Some decoctions may separate when cooled. Straining the plant parts while the mixture is hot allows you to retain the compounds. You may want to wear gloves and squeeze the excess fluids from the plant parts to reduce loss.

Since decoctions tend to be stronger than infusions because of the evaporation of some of the liquids, you will use less at a time. You can store extra liquids from your decoction in the refrigerator, often for 2-3 days depending on the plants that you have selected. You will want to store the decoction in a safe container like a stainless steel or glass bottle. Allow the mixture to cool before storage.

Shake or stir the decoction before each use. This ensures that any compounds that have separated are re-distributed.

Syrup

A decoction or infusion can sometimes be bitter or more liquid in nature than the treatment requires so it is a common practice to make it into syrup. Syrups are especially useful when dosing will be by the teaspoon or tablespoon instead of by the cup. Making an infusion or decoction into syrup may also help to extend the shelf life.

The amount of sweetener product like Agave, sugar, or honey used to make syrup will vary depending on the personal preference of the user.

Traditional syrup is made using about 8 ounces of herbal fluid to 4 ounces of liquid honey, sweetener, or sugar. This amount will vary depending on personal preference and type of sweetener being used.

Heat the sweetener you have selected until it becomes liquefied. Remove the sweetener from the heat and add the plant infusion, powder, or decoction. Blend the ingredients well.

You may want to alter the mixture depending on the eventual use of the syrup. The thicker the syrup the better it "sticks". An example of a time when you want syrup to adhere well is if the syrup will be used as a treatment for a sore throat.

When you have attained the consistency you want, pour the finished syrup into a sterile, dark container. Refrigerating the syrup will help to extend the shelf life further. You can also add a natural preservative if you wish but research any preservatives carefully because some may interfere with or even destroy the beneficial compounds of the syrup. Typical syrup will keep usable for between 8 to 16 weeks.

Electuary

The terms electuaries and syrups are used interchangeably by some people but are actually two different products. An electuary is a paste made of powdered plant products mixed with a base.

Powdered plant products are traditionally mixed with sweeteners like syrup, honey, berry jam or sugar and water. The powders and base are blended to make a paste. A paste is thicker than syrup.

The plant products used to make an electuary should be powdered as finely as possible. A coffee grinder, food processor, or mortar and pestle all work well for powdering dried plant parts.

The composition of an electuary can be as basic as one part powdered plant product mixed with two parts honey and as complex as dozens of types of plant product mixed with multiple sweetening agents and carriers. Honey is a good choice as a base for many people since it can actually help to extend the usable life of the finished product. The powdered plants that are used will depend entirely on the supplement you need. You can use as few or many plant powders and you want when making an electuary.

You will want to vary the balances of powder to carrier agent to suit your needs. Some powders are heavier and will require more carriers while others are lighter, and will need less. Common electuaries can range from 1 part powder to 3 parts carrier to 1 part powder to ½-part carrier.

When you have all of your components measured, heat the carrier or base slightly and blend in the powdered herbs. Store an unused electuary in a sterile, glass or metal container with a tight fitting lid.

Extracts

An extract is a product made by separating the active compounds of a plant into a condensed state. Extraction is traditionally accomplished using a solvent, expressing the compounds, or reducing a decoction to a thickened state.

Alcohol Extract or Tincture
An extract or tincture is made using plant parts and a solvent. Common solvents are grain alcohol, vodka, or wine. A simple explanation of the differences between extracts and tinctures is that an extract is traditionally made using 1 part plant matter to 1 part liquid while a tincture is made using 1 part plant matter to 3, 4, or even 5 parts liquid.

Alcohol extracts require three basic ingredients. You will need a glass or ceramic jar with a tightly fitting lid, a solvent like alcohol, and the desired plant products.

You will harvest and clean the plant parts according to the standard harvesting practices. Cut the plant parts into finely chopped pieces. You can use a blender or food processor to chop the plant parts. Make certain you do not grind them into such fine pieces you cannot strain the plant parts from the liquid when your extract is complete.

Place the plant parts into the jar. Fill the jar with the selected alcohol, making certain all of the plant parts are covered.

There are commercially and traditionally established ratios of alcohol, water, and plant materials for each type of plant you might process. You can refer to specific entries for the particular plant product or to commercial preparation standards to determine what is best for the particular plant you are extracting. In general, the higher the oil contents of the plant material, the higher the alcohol necessary to extract the beneficial compounds.

Once the jar is filled, seal the jar. Shake the jar to agitate the materials and to ensure that as much of the plant product is in contact with the alcohol as possible. Place the jar in a cool, dark place where it will not be disturbed. Every morning and night, shake the jar to agitate the mixture and distribute the plant parts in the alcohol.

The amount of time you will need to make an extract depends on the type of plant materials you are using. Soft leaves and petals yield more quickly than hard seeds & barks. Most extracts take between 2 and 8 weeks.

The final content of the alcohol extract should be approximately 25% alcohol. This helps to inhibit bacterial and fungal growth. Bacteria and fungus will still grow in an alcohol tincture but this ratio helps to slow the process.

When the extract has reached the strength you want, strain the plant products out of the liquid. You will want to squeeze all of the fluid out of the plant materials.

Alcohol extracts and tinctures should be stored away from light.

You can use a preservative to extend the shelf life of your tincture though it is not necessary. Some plant parts are natural preservatives.

Finished alcohol extracts or tinctures should be stored in dark glass containers to prevent the loss of active compounds. A finished alcohol extract will keep for as much as 3 years.

Expressed Extract

You can make an expressed extract by pressing the juice out of certain types of plant parts. Not all plants can be juiced. If you are working with a plant part that can be juiced, you will express the liquid using a plant press, juicer, or simply by squeezing the applicable part.

Some juices can be used as a remedy in their own right. You will want to save every usable part of the plants you buy, grow, or harvest.

Typical extract treatments would use the plant part that is left after the excess juices are expressed. You will apply the plant parts to the affected area or prepare it according to the supplement instructions for ingestion.

Simmer Extract

Some extracts are made through simmering. Much like a decoction, you will simmer the plant parts to condense the beneficial compounds down to their most potent form. Extracts can be made using oil, alcohol, vinegar, or water. You will follow the same steps as you do when making a decoction but you will reduce the fluid to ¼ or less of its original liquid volume. In other words, if you start with 1 cup of fluid, you will finish when you have ¼ cup or less of fluid.

Infusion Flavoring

Sometimes the flavor of liquids like vinegar, oils, and alcohol can be enhanced by the addition of plant parts. Infusion flavorings provide not only the flavor and aroma but also the compounds of the plant parts selected for the process.

Alcohol Infusion

Flavored alcohol has become very popular in recent years. You can make your own flavored, custom blends at home and add beneficial compounds customized to your specific wants & needs.

You can make flavored alcohol infusions using the same barks, flowers, fruits & leaves that you use to make your other products. Many available recipes include popular flavor combinations. You can use these if you just want to make flavored cocktails. Since this is all about obtaining the benefits of plant products, you may want to experiment with your own custom blends that not only taste great but also provide the healthy supplemental benefits that suit your personal situation.

You can make an alcohol infusion out of almost any liquor but most people prefer vodka. Vodka has a neutral flavor that can easily be changed through plant infusions. Rum, gin, whiskey, almost any alcohol you prefer will take flavor from a plant infusion. Select the alcohol that suits your preferences.

The biggest difference in this type of infusion is that fresh flowers, fruits, leaves, and other parts work better than the dried variety when making a flavored infusion. You will clean the plant parts you have selected. You should remove any damaged or spoiled pieces. You will also want to remove and discard any plant parts you do not want in your final product. For example, if you are using berries as part of your mixture, you may want to remove any leaves and stems attached to the berry. These will have different properties and give the final infusion a different taste.

You will need to chop or grind the plant parts. The finer you chop the plant parts, the better the flavor will infuse. Unless you are using the plant parts as a dressing, you will not want to chop them so fine that they are difficult to remove from the finished product.

The amount of plant parts to alcohol you are using, the exact plant parts you select, and the flavor you want from your finished product all influence the ratio of plant to alcohol you will use. A good guideline is ½ part plant parts to 1 part alcohol. You can adjust this as you become more familiar with the flavors of the plant parts you select.

Since this instructional is not dealing with very specific ingredients but rather generalities of processes, it is impossible to predict exactly what the balance will be for your particular recipe. Some plant products like juicy fruits yield flavor more quickly than some tougher plant products like nuts. You may need more or less alcohol to extract the flavor depending on exactly what you are using and how you want your drink to taste.

When you feel the mix you have created is likely to yield the strength and flavor you desire, seal the infusion jar with a tight fitting lid and place it in a warm area of your home. Some people find that the flavor infuses more quickly when the jar is placed in a sunny location. This may lower the beneficial effects of the plant compound but since flavored alcohol is as much about taste as it is about benefits, you may want to consider using sunlight as a tool. A more pure method of infusing is to keep light away from the mixture to help protect as many of the beneficial compounds as possible.

No matter what plant products you are using as a flavoring, you will want to keep a close taste watch on your infusion. The flavor is going to be custom suited to your tastes and needs so sample a few drops of the infusion every couple of days. When the flavor mix reaches your preference, the infusion is done. If the flavor mix becomes too strong, you can always dilute it with extra alcohol.

After your flavor has reached its peak, you will strain the plant parts from the alcohol base. A coffee filter, cheesecloth, or fine kitchen strainer all work well for removing plant parts.

Store the liquid in a clean, airtight container and enjoy. Just remember that you have transferred the active compounds of the plant parts into your alcohol and read the maximum daily limits and potential side effects before using your new product.

Vinegar Infusion

Many people enjoy the flavor and aroma of a custom vinegar blend.   Flavored vinegars are made following the same processes as flavored alcohol. You simply replace the alcohol with vinegar.

There are two important considerations regarding infused vinegar that you should remember. The vinegar will contain the compounds of the plants used during the process. Most people tend to use vinegar more freely in the family diet than they do alcohol. You should always review the potential effects, good and bad, of any plant materials before adding them to your diet. The infused vinegar will also be prone to the same type of spoilage as any other vinegar product.

OILS

Oil extracts, oil flavorings, and essential oils are very different products. Each of them can be made at home but they do require slightly different processes.   The processes for aromatic, supplement, and flavored oils are similar to making other supplements & flavorings. The differences between one method of extraction and the next is the strength of the finished product.

Cold Oil Infusion

An oil infusion is used to extract the oil soluble compounds in plant parts for use as a flavoring, aroma element, and supplement product.

You can infuse oil using the same processes you would use for alcohol and vinegar flavorings. You will harvest, clean, and prepare the plant parts you want in your oil according to the standard harvest instructions. Many people find that dried plant parts work better in oil infusions than fresh plant parts. Dried plant parts have had most of the water removed from the plant and may blend with oils better than fresh plants.

You should select the oils that work best for your personal situation and your taste preference. Olive oil is the most commonly selected flavored oil base but other oils work equally well. If you will be using your oil as a supplement instead of a flavoring, you will want to modify the oil selection accordingly. If you are planning to use the finished product in a topical treatment, jojoba oil is a nice choice. You should spend some time considering the uses you plan for your finished product and research the best oils for your purposes.

When making the oil infusion, follow the alcohol infusion instructions but replace the alcohol with oil. Just like with any infusion, it is important to remember that the oil will contain the active compounds of the plant parts you selected. Make certain you use oil according to the correct daily dosing limits and consider the potential effects of the plant parts before serving the oil product to others.

Sun Oil Bath

One of the most common methods of extracting essential oils from a plant is to use an oil bath. You will select the plant materials to be used. Chop them into fine pieces. Place the chopped materials in a glass jar. Add a carrier oil with a long shelf life like jojoba until the plant matter is completely covered. Seal the jar and place it in the sun.

Direct sunlight may heat the oils too much so you should select an area that receives diffused sunlight. Windowsills are the most commonly chosen location. Allow the oil bath to heat throughout the day. Shake the jar each night to speed the process.

Continue to allow the oil bath to extract the essence until you feel that no further progress is being made. Strain the plant materials out of the oils. The resulting oil will not be as strong as the oils you obtain through distillation or solvent extraction.

You can re-infuse the oils to make them stronger. Simply repeat the process using the same oils as you did during the first sunbath but use fresh plant products. Each time you repeat the process with the same oil, the resulting product will be stronger.

The stronger the oil becomes, the higher the likelihood of a reaction. You should make sure you protect your skin from the oils and plant parts to minimize the likelihood of irritation and have a comprehensive understanding of the maximum dosage and effects of any plants you used in your bath.

Using Infused Oils

Infused oils are frequently used in culinary and supplemental preparations. Infused oils are also used to make lotions, creams, and other topical preparations. You can find a variety of natural product recipes for the hair, lips, nails and skin. The infused oils you have made using the appropriate plant parts can be used in replacement for the liquid in your selected recipe.

There are two important considerations regarding infused oils you should remember. The oils will contain the compounds of the plants used during the process. You should always review the potential effects, good and bad, of any plant materials before adding them to your diet or personal care products. You should also remember that products made with infused oils will be prone to the same type of spoilage as any other oil product.

Essential Oils

An essential oil is much stronger than infused oil. When you make an infusion, you are diluting the compounds with the alcohol, vinegar, or oil base. When making an essential oil, you are capturing the concentrated plant essences in their pure form and not diluting the results.

Essential oils are most frequently used for topical and aromatherapy treatments. Essential oils are often very powerful and should not be applied directly to the skin. Essential oils must be diluted before use.

The method of extraction you use to garner essential oils will depend on the specific plant, ultimate use, and desired strength of the oil.

Distillation

The most common method of commercial essential oil extraction is by distillation. Distillation uses water to help extract the oils. There are different methods of distillation. You can purchase a distillation unit for personal use, make your own distillation unit using a pressure cooker and tubing, or you can use one of the more common home methods of extraction like solvents.

Steam Distillation

Steam distillation uses a source of steam piped into the distillation unit at a high pressure. The steam passes through the plant material and exits into a condenser unit. The product in the condenser unit is the plant essence or essential oil.

Steam distillation units can be purchased or you can make your own steam distillation unit from a pressure cooker, tubing, and capture jar. These unites are somewhat complex and you will want to review commercial distillation units and homemade distillation unit creation instructions before attempting to make a unit of your own.

Hydro-Distillation

Hydro-distillation is extraction accomplished by covering plant materials in water. You can envision it as being similar to making a soup. The water is heated to produce a steam that contains the plant essence. The steam is captured and used in therapeutics. This method works well for tougher materials like nuts, wood, and roots.

Hydro-distillation units are similar to standard steam distillation units and can be purchased for in home use. There are also many instructions available free on the internet that tell you how to make your own hydro-distillation unit.

Tray Distillation

Tray distillation is much like the process you would use to steam vegetables for food. The plant material is placed into a sieve like pan. The sieve is then placed over another pan filled with water. A tightly fitting lid with a tube leading out of it is placed on top. The water is boiled so the steam passes through the plant material. The steam extracts the oils from the plant and carries it upward to the tube. The tube captures the concentrated liquid and pipes it to a holding unit. This method of distillation works best for soft plant materials. These units are also available for purchase or can be made following some simple instructions available free through an internet search.

Simmer Extraction

You can simmer extract compounds from plant products. This method of extraction does use more heat and runs the danger of destroying the very compounds you want to protect, but it is a quick and simple method of extracting essential oils at home.

You will select the base oil you want to use for your simmer. The type of oil you select will depend largely on the ultimate use you will make of your essential oils. If you are using the oils in skin care, massage treatments, or other topical preparations then you will want to select oil that is compatible with your skin type. Jojoba oil is often a good choice if you are unsure of what oils will work well for you because it is similar to the body's own natural oils. If you will use your oils in aromatherapy treatments, you will want to select neutral oil that diffuses well.

Prepare your plant materials by chopping, grinding, or pounding the plant parts. Once again, the more parts of the plant you expose to the oils, the better the extraction results you will achieve.

Put the prepared plant parts in the pot you will use for heating. Some people like to use a crock-pot while others prefer to use a saucepan. Either will yield approximately the same results so the choice is a matter of personal preference.

Add enough of the selected carrier oil to cover the plant materials.

Cover the pan with a tight fitting lid.

Most people find they have better results and improve the likelihood of success if they use a water bath to heat the oils. Select a pan that is larger and deeper than the pan you have chosen for your plant & oil mixture. Fill this pan with 2-3 inches of water. Place the plant & oil pan into the water bath pan.

Heat the oil and plant mixture to a temperature between 100° and 125°. Do not overheat the oil bath because you will cook the plants instead of extracting the compounds.

Allow the mixture to simmer for 3 to 4 hours, stirring occasionally. You should take care not to reduce the oil amount when you stir the plants by allowing oils to escape. You want to minimize evaporation.

When you mixture has finished simmering, remove it from the heat source. You can strain the plant materials from the oil immediately or allow the plant & oil mixture to continue to steep. Some plants can steep for weeks and retain some active compounds while others will yield all of the available compounds during the heating process. You will need to get to know the plant materials you have selected in order to decide when you have extracted the maximum benefit from the plant. It is important to experiment to learn how the plant parts will react to different processes. Generally, the softer the plant materials, the more quickly they yield the compounds.

It is recommended that you use rubber gloves to protect your skin when working with essential oils. The stronger the essential oils, the more likely they are to cause a reaction.

Strain the oils through cheesecloth. Squeeze any remaining oil out of the plant materials. Discard the leftover plant materials.

You can repeat the process with new plant materials and the oil you gathered from the first extraction. Each repeated extraction with the same oil will increase the potency of the finished product.

Solvent Extraction

Some plant essences cannot survive the heat distillation methods. These will require cold extraction. You can use a solvent to extract essential oils through cold methods.

Select the plant materials that contain the highest amount of active scent compounds. Chop, grind, or bruise the materials as appropriate for the types of plant parts you have selected. Place the chopped and bruised plant material on a tray with perforations. A dehydrator tray works well. Place the tray over a capture pan.

You will use a solvent like grain alcohol or hexane to extract matter from the plant. The solvent will extract everything that is dissolvable in the plant including waxes, pigments, and the aromatic oils.

You can use the solvent as a wash. To do this, you must have a capture pan that sits below the perforated plant tray. Pour the solvent over the plant materials. Remove the resulting liquid from the capture tray and pour it over the plant products again. Continue this process until the wash produces little or no new extraction.

You can also use the solvent as a bath. To do this, you must have a capture pan that allows the perforated tray to sit inside of it. Place the plant materials on the perforated tray. Sit the tray inside the capture pan. Pour the solvent over the plants until they are just covered. Allow the bath to sit, stirring occasionally. The length of time you must allow the bath to sit will depend on the plant material. Each plant material will give up the essences at a different pace. You can agitate the plant product occasionally to speed the process. When you believe that there is no longer any matter left to be extracted, remove the plant materials from the bath. Strain any remaining solid matter from the liquid.

When you have removed the solid matter, place the liquid into a container and seal it. The liquid should not completely fill the container. You should keep at least ¼ of the space in the container empty to allow for expansion.

Allow the mixture to rest for a day or two. You will note that the materials separate. You should be able to view three layers.

You will have an opaque or thick layer of impurities. This layer will either fall to the bottom of the jar or lay on the top of the mixture.

The solvent alcohol will appear neutral.

You will see a layer that contains the oil essences. This layer will not appear as polluted as the impurity layer or as clear as the alcohol layer. This is your essential oil layer.

When your layers have formed, carefully lift the jar without agitating the layers. Loosen the lid to prevent breakage as the materials expand. Place the jar in the freezer. The oils and impurities will freeze. The alcohol will not freeze.

Place the entire frozen mass on a straining board. If the materials have frozen to the jar, you can gently separate them with a stainless steel knife.

The alcohol will drain away. Capture the alcohol in another jar as it strains away. You will want to freeze the alcohol again to gather any remaining oils that did not separate during the first freeze.

If the oils and impure layer are next to each other, use a knife to separate the usable oils from the impurities. Discard the impurities.

Place the frozen mass of oils onto a cheesecloth spread over a capture bowl or jar. As the mixture thaws, the oils will strain into the bowl. Anything that remains in the cheesecloth is plant material that was missed during the first straining. This can be discarded. The oils that strain into the bowl are the essential oils. Place the finished essential oils into your final storage jars.

The alcohol that you set aside earlier should be returned to the freezer for a second time. Any oils that remain in the solvent will freeze.

When the oils have frozen, remove the jar from the freezer and strain it through cheesecloth spread over an empty capture bowl. The alcohol will drain through the cheesecloth leaving the frozen oil behind. You can discard the alcohol or save it for use in your next extraction. Do not use the alcohol to extract the oils from a different type of plant material unless you have considered the active compounds of both types of plant materials.

The frozen oil parts should be allowed to thaw into another jar. The cheesecloth will filter any residual plant solids that remain. Add the captured oils to the essential oil jar you created during the first separation.

Store the essential oils in a cool, dark area for maximum shelf life.

Cold Pressing
Cold pressing works well for citrus peels and other plant parts whose oils can be released by scoring the plant product. You will score the plant, press the body and capture the oils being released.

External Use of Plant Products

Many plant products are used in traditional topical preparations. There are numerous ways of using plant products in external preparations. You can use plant products in cleaners, washes, ointments, salves, creams, poultices, lotions and so forth. Almost any topical preparation you purchase at the store can be made from scratch using natural ingredients.

There are numerous natural product recipe guides available, including my Green & Natural book series that include simple recipes that you can create to replace almost every product you use. You can also create your own custom topical preparations using the plants detailed in the compendium.

The following explanations will help you to gain a fundamental picture of some of the most common topical preparations and the steps necessary to create them yourself.

Fomentation & Compress

A fomentation is the external use of strong herbal infusions.

If you are using soft plant parts, you will follow the infusion instructions but allow the plant parts to steep for a longer period than you would when creating a drinkable infusion.

If you are using hard plant parts, you will follow the instructions from making a decoction but reduce the fluid to 1/3 or even ¼ of the original fluid amount.

Once the infusion or decoction has reached the desired strength, you will soak a clean cloth in the liquid. Cotton and wool are common fabric choices for fomentations. The saturated cloth is then applied to the affected part.

You should use most fomentations while they are still hot. In general, you want the fomentation to be as hot as can be handled. When the cloth cools, saturate it in the fluid again and reapply it to the affected area. You may want to use two cloths. One is applied while the other is soaking in the hot liquid.

Most fomentations can be wrapped in clean plastic and an elastic bandage to help retain the heat and to keep moisture from getting all over everything nearby. The clean plastic should be on the outside of the fomentation, not the area that will touch your body.

You will continue to apply the fomentation according to the instructions of the plant parts you are using and condition you are treating. The time usage of a fomentation could range from less than an hour to a couple of days. Gently re-heat the fomentation when it becomes too cool to use.

Some conditions do not lend themselves to heat. If the patient, condition, or other reason makes hot heat undesirable, the fluid can be used as a cool compress. You will follow the same instructions as you would when making a fomentation, but you will allow the mixture to cool before applying it to the skin. When the compress becomes too warm, you will exchange it for a fresh, cool cloth.

Poultice

A poultice is made by chopping, bruising, or grating plant parts into smaller parts and applying them directly to an injured, inflamed, or problem area. The size of the plant parts used will vary depending on the instructions relating to the specific plant, malady, and treatment.

Some poultices are made by cutting the plant so that the internal parts are exposed and applying the product directly to the skin. An example of this type of poultice is the use of an aloe leaf to sooth a burn.

Other poultice recommendations require you to nearly powder the plant parts and mix the product with a small amount of water to form a paste.

The method of application will depend on the plant product and condition you are trying to alleviate.

Some poultices are hot preparations. A hot poultice is most often used to increase blood flow, alleviate pain, reduce inflammation, and relax muscles.

Hot poultices can be made by adding hot water to the ground plant parts to form a paste and applying the paste to the affected area.

A few plant parts should be directly heated before applying them to the area to be treated. You should use caution when heating plant parts because overheating can destroy beneficial compounds.

The most common method of making a hot poultice is to layer the plant parts on the area to be treated and then cover the area with a moist, hot cloth. This application method helps to increase the heat and lengthen the time of the treatment. The cloth is moistened and heated, usually using the microwave or the steam from a pan of boiling water. The cloth is exchanged for a warm one as it cools.

Some poultices are cold preparations. Cold poultices are traditionally used to draw heat or toxins from an area, reduce congestion, and as a counter to hot poultices in cases of painful inflammation. Common uses of a cold poultice are in treating skin sores, ulcers, wounds, and skin conditions like eczema.

When creating a cold poultice, you will wet the plant parts with room temperature to icy cold fluid as indicated by the plant parts being used and condition being treated. The cold compress is then applied directly to the area being treated.

Poultices occasionally call for a plant part that is irritating to the skin. If the necessary plant parts include skin irritants, you should use a thin layer of cloth between the skin and the poultice. This will not allow for concentrated absorption of beneficial compounds but it will protect the skin from damage while still providing some benefit.

It is important to remember that using plant parts as a topical preparation still delivers the compounds of the plant into the body. The skin is the largest organ in the body and it readily absorbs compounds that are placed into direct contact with it. You can overuse a poultice.

Ointment

An ointment is made by blending powdered plant parts, plant decoctions, plant extracts, or plant oils into a base. Ointments generally contain oils, thickeners, hardeners, and plant parts. Ointments do not usually contain water.

When making ointments you will need a base, the preferred plant parts, and sterile containers. You may also choose to use a thickening agent, hardener, and preservative depending on the type of application, storage length, and slip desired in the product.

The base or carrier can be a liquid substance like almond oil, jojoba, or Vitamin E oil or semi liquid like cocoa butter or lanolin. These carriers each have properties, benefits and side effects of their own. You will want to consider the potential effects of the carrier when making your selection.

The oily, liquid carriers are commonly used in massage lotions and for creating topical pain-relief rubs. These can be made into a thicker ointment by incorporating a thickening agent and a hardener into the recipe.

The semi-solid carriers like cocoa butter tend to be used in products meant for application in a thin layer like in skin conditioning preparations. These can still be blended with thickening agents and hardeners but it is often not necessary.

Depending on the use of your finished product, the recipe may benefit from a hardener. The need for a hardener depends on the application method you plan for your product. The most common hardeners are waxes like beeswax and paraffin wax.

Some ointments will be used very quickly and are designed to treat a short-term issue. Others may be used over a period of weeks or months. If you plan to use the ointment over a period of weeks, you will want to add a preservative. Some plants have natural preservative properties while others will require enhancement. You should review the compendium to decide what type of preservative will work best with your particular recipe.

Most ointments are oil based. You will want select the appropriate oil base for your particular need. You will also find that using powdered or oil extracted plant components makes blending the ointment easier. Water based extractions or infusions do not blend as easily and may require the additional of an emulsifier.

Use a water bath to heat any carrier oil, thickening agents and hardener you plan to incorporate into your recipe. You should not heat the plant parts because heat may destroy the beneficial components.

When the carrier oil, thickener and hardening agents are warmed to a liquid state, whip them into the plant materials you have prepared and then immediately pour the resulting mixture into a clean tub, jar, or tube.

Seal the filled container and add the appropriate label.

Depending on the exact ingredients you have used, you may need to shake the mixture before each use to re-blend the ingredients. Ointments that contain thickeners and hardeners will not need to be shaken as much as those that do not.

Labeling
If you are only making one type of plant product, you will probably remember what is in the jar or bag, but chances are good you will not be able to stop with just one product. Once you realize how easy and satisfying making your own natural products can be, you will probably make many different products intended for many different uses, making labeling an important part of the process.

There is certain information that I find invaluable

Date Started
Plants Included
Plant parts used
Amount
Base – oils, alcohol, vinegar, etc
Amount
Date Completed – Storage Date
Expiration Date

You will want to continue to explore the many, many uses of plant products. This guide gives you a wide range of products you can make and use today. My compendium provides an in-depth look at a larger variety of traditional plants used by herbalists. Scientific and natural research is constantly being done to fine tune our knowledge of the potential of plants. There are many, many sources of plant knowledge, recipes, and product creation guides available. I hope that this guide has given you a healthy knowledge base and a basic understanding of the potential uses of the plants you see every day. Feel free to drop me a note telling me about your new discoveries, recipes you love, or just to say hi! There is nothing more satisfying than sharing my love of plants and nature with a fellow creator.

Glossary

Abortifacient – A substance that is capable of inducing an abortion

Adoptogenic – A substance that has a normalize effect against changes brought about by stressors

Acid – A chemical that produces a pH of less than 7 in water. Having a low pH.

Adjective - Adjective dyes are those dyes that require use of a mordant to bind the color to the fiber.

Alkali – A chemical that produces a pH of more than 7. Having a high pH.

Alopecia – Baldness. The partial or complete loss of hair.

Alum (aluminum sulfate) - Alum is a naturally occurring basic mordant.

Alum (aluminum acetate) - A naturally occurring common mordant.

Amenorrhea – Absence of menstruation.

Analgesic - A pain-killing drug or medicine.

Aniline - Aniline dyes or basic dyes are a class of synthetic dyes derived from coal tar that produce brilliant colors but poor colorfastness.

Anodyne - A pain-killing drug or medicine.

Antibacterial – A substance that is active against bacteria.

Anticonvulsant – A substance used to reduce or prevent convulsions

Anti-emetic - A substance that reduces or prevents nausea or vomiting.

Antifungal – A substance that is used to alleviate or prevent fungal infections.

Antihistamine - A substance that inhibits the physiological effects of histamine. A histamine is the chemical released by the body during an allergic reaction.

Anti-Inflammatory – A substance used to reduce inflammation.

Anti-Microbial- A substance that kills or inhibits the growth of microorganisms

Anti-Oxidant – Molecule that inhibits the oxidation of other molecules.

Anti-Periodic – A substance used to treat malarial-type symptoms or to prevent the recurrence of malarial like symptoms.

Anti-Parasitic – A substance used to treat or prevent parasitic infestations.

Anti-Septic – A substance capable of preventing or treating infection by inhibiting the growth of microorganisms.

Anti-Spasmodic - A substance that suppresses muscle spasms.

Antitussive – A substance used to suppress or relieve coughing.

Anti-Viral – A substance that prevents or treats viral infections by killing a virus or that suppresses its ability to replicate.

Aphrodisiac – A substance that stimulates sexual desire.

Aromatic – A substance having a pleasant and distinctive smell that is used as a treatment.

Aroma Therapy – Aromatic plant extracts or essential oils to cause a physical or psychological effect in treatments.

Aspergillus - A type of common molds that cause food spoilage and potentially disease.

Astringent - Substance that causes the contraction of body tissues.

Bleeding – Color rinsing out of a dyed textile.

Botanical Name – The Latin name give to a species of plant to distinguish it from other plants.

Bursitis – A condition where there is inflammation in the bursa – elbow, knee, shoulder.

Cardiac - Relating to the heart

Carminative – Substance that relieves flatulence.

Cathartic - A purgative substance.

Chalogogue - A substance that stimulates the secretion of bile from the gallbaldder.

Chrome – (Potassium Dichromate) Chrome is a naturally occurring common mordant.
Citric Acid – Acid found in many plant products but most common to citrus fruits. Citric Acid is used to neutralize high pH.

Coagulant - A substance that causes blood to clot or coagulate

Colorant - Substance that colors something usually food, cosmetics, or textile products.

Colorfastness – A measure of how resistant a dye material is to fading.

Common Name – The non-specific name used for everyday reference to a plant

Comminution – The action of reducing a material or substance. When processing plants the act of reducing the size of the plant parts by cutting, grinding, or pounding

Conjunctivitis – An infection or irritation causing inflammation, itching, and redness of the white part of the eye.

COPD – Chronic Obstructive Pulmonary Disease involving constriction of the airways and difficulty breathing.

Copper (copper sulphate) – Copper is a naturally occurring mordant used to give green casts to textiles.

Copperas – Term used for iron ore (ferrous sulfate) used to depress the colors of a dye bath.

Cream of Tarter (potassium bitartrate) - A naturally occurring color modifier. Cream of Tarter is not a stand-alone mordant but acts in tandem with other mordants.

Decoction – The result of concentration the essence of a substance or plant part by heating or boiling.

Demulcent – A substance that soothes inflammation and protects irritated internal tissues.

Depurative – Substance that facilitates the removal of impurities or cleansing of bodily fluids.

Detoxification - Process of removing toxic substances or qualities from matter.

Diaphoretic – A substance that induces perspiration.

Digestive –

Diosgenin – A steroid compound used in the synthesis of steroid hormones.

Diuretic – A substance causing increased passing of urine.

Dram – A unit of measurement equaling approximately 1/16 of a dry weigth ounce in US measurement 1/8 of a fluid ounce in Apothecary measurement.

Dye – Color-bearing organic compounds that penetrate fiber or other matter.

Dyebath – A solution of colorant and water used to color textiles.

Dyestuff – Any raw material that releases dye.

Dysmenorrheal – Menstruation with excessive pain involving abdominal and lower back cramping.

Emetic - Substance that causes vomiting.

Emmenagogue – Substance that stimulates or increases menstrual flow.

Emollient – Substance that has a softening or soothing affect on the skin.

Estrogenic – A substance acting like, relating to, or caused by estrogen.

Expectorant – A substance that promotes the secretion of mucus from the air passages.

Expression - The process of forcibly separating liquids from solids.

Febrifuge – Substance used to reduce fever.

Fluid extract – A type of fluid-solid substance obtained from plant matter through water or alcohol processing

Fugitive Color – Color that is prone to fading when exposed to sunlight or washing.

Galactogogue - Substance that stimulates milk secretion.

Glycosides – A compound formed from a simple sugar and another compound by the replacement of a hydroxyl in the sugar molecule.

Gram-Positive Bacteria – A class of bacterial that are stained dark blue or violet by gram staining including bacteria such as pneumococci, staphylococci, and strepotcocci.

Gram Negative Bacteria - A class of bacterial that do not retain the stain used in gram staining including bacteria such as e. coli, shingella, salmonella.

Hallucinogenic – A psychoactive substance capable of producing hallucinations or altered sensory experiences.

Hepatic - Of or relating to the liver.

Hydration - The process of combining with or giving water.

Hypoallergenic – A substance unlikely to cause an allergic reaction.

Hypoglycemic – A condition indicated by low blood sugar.

Hypotensive – A condition of abnormally low blood pressure.

Histamine - The chemical released by the body during an allergic reaction.

Immunostimulant - Substance that stimulate the immune system to fight infection.

Infusion – Aqueous – A drink or extract made by soaking plant parts in water.

Infusion – Oil – A drink, extract, or product made by soaking plant parts in oil.

Insecticide - Substance used for killing insects.

Interferon - A protein released in response to a virus that has the ability to inhibit virus reproduction.

Iron Ore (ferrous sulfate) used to mute or darken the colors of a dye bath.

Laxative – Substance that stimulates or facilitates evacuation of the bowels

Lighfastness - A measure of a dye products resistance to fading from light exposure.

Lipase – An enzyme that facilitates the breakdown of fats to fatty acids and glycol to other alcohols.

Lye (sodium hydroxide) – A caustic substance used to shift pH.

Maceration – Softening plant materials by soaking or steeping in a liquid. To separate the compounds by soaking or steeping

Menorrhagia – Abnormally heavy menstrual bleeding.

Menstruum - A solvent or mix of solvents.

Microphage – A cell found in the tissues or at the site of an infection that takes in foreign material.

Mordant – A substance that combines with a dye or stain to fix the colorant into a material.

Muscle Relaxant – A substance that reduces muscle tone or contractibility.

Narcotic – A psychoactive substance affecting mood or behavior.

Natural Dye – Dye derived from animal, mineral, or plant matter.

Natural Fiber – A fiber obtained from an animal, mineral, or plant source.

Nervine – A psychoactive substance that calms the nerves.

Nutritive – Substance that providing nourishment; nutritious.

Over Dye – The act of placing one dye over another to alter the finished tone.

Percolation - The extraction of soluble components by passing the liquid through a filtering medium.

pH – A scale for measuring the acidity or alkalinity of a substance. A pH of 7 is neutral. Low pH is acidic. High pH is alkaline.

Pharynx   The membrane lined cavity behind the nose and mouth that connects them to the esophagus.

Phytoestrogen - Compounds found in plants that can mimic the effects of estrogen.

Pleurae – The membranes lining the thorax and enveloping the lungs.

Pleurisy – An inflammation of the pleurae that causes pain when breathing.

Polysaccharide – A carbohydrate that is a compound of sugar molecules bonded together.

Proof Spirit – A mixture of alcohol and water containing 50% alcohol by volume standard in the US.

Purgative – A substance that is strongly laxative in effect.

Pulmonary – Relating to the pulmonary system.

Phytosterol – A group of naturally occurring steroid plant compounds.

Reactive Dye – A class of synthetic dyes that are used to dye natural fibers that traditionally resist taking color.

Reparative – A substance that helps to repair.

Rhinitis – Inflammation of the mucus membrane of the nose.

Rubefacient – A substance whose external application produces increased circulation or redness of the skin.

Saponins – A class of steroid and terpenoid glycosides that are used in detergents and foam when shaken with water.

Sciatica – Nerve pain caused by compression of a spinal nerve in the lower back that affects the back, hip, or leg.

Sedative – Substance that causes a calming or sleep-inducing effect.

Squalene – An oily liquid that is the precursor to sterols.

Sterols – Naturally occurring unsaturated steroid alcohols.

Steroidal - Relating to steroid hormones or their effects.

Stimulant – A substance that raises levels of physiological or nervous activity in the body.

Styptic – A substance that causes bleeding to stop.

Substantive Dyes – Dyes that produce lasting color without the use of a mordant.

Succus – The juice several liquids in the body commonly termed digestive juices but also the juice of fresh plant material.

Sudorific – Relating to or causing sweating.

Tannin – A naturally occurring component of some plant products used as a mordant. It aids some dyes in being self-mordanting and shifts colors to a browner tone.

Tin (stannous chloride) - A metallic salt used as a brightening mordant.

Tincture – A substance made by dissolving plant materials in alcohol.

Vasodilator – Substance that causes dilation of blood vessels.

Vermifuge – Substance that destroys parasites.

Viscosity – The resistance of a liquid to movement and flow.

Washfastness - A measure of how resistant a dye product is to fading over time due to exposure to water or soap.

References

Full reference list from a compendium of beneficial herbs and oils.

Personal observations, experimentations, and family notes Laurie Pippen

A. Abdul Rahuman, Geetha Gopalakrishnan, P. Venkatesan and Kannappan Geetha (2008). "Isolation and identification of mosquito larvicidal compound from Abutilon indicum (Linn.) Sweet". Parasitology Research 102

A. Ngan & R. Conduit (2011). "A double-blind, placebo-controlled investigation of the effects of Passiflora incarnata (passionflower) herbal tea on subjective sleep quality". Phytotherapy Research 25

Abbott, I. A. (1996). Ethnobotany of seaweeds: clues to uses of seaweeds. Hydrobiologia.

Adhami, VM; Aziz, MH; Mukhtar, H; Ahmad, N (2003). "Activation of prodeath Bcl-2 family proteins and mitochondrial apoptosis pathway by sanguinarine in immortalized human HaCaT keratinocytes". Clinical cancer research 9

Agrawal, K. (1992). Biochemical pharmacology of blood and bloodforming organs. Berlin: Springer-Verlag.

Agarwal R, Gupta SK, Agrawal SS, Srivastava S, Saxena R (2008). "Oculohypotensive effects of foeniculum vulgare in experimental models of glaucoma". Indian J. Physiol. Pharmacol. 52

Ahmad, Nihal; Gupta, Sanjay; Husain, Mirza M.; Heiskanen, Kaisa M.; Mukhtar, Hasan (2000). "Differential Antiproliferative and Apoptotic Response of Sanguinarine for Cancer Cells versus Normal Cells". Clinical Cancer Research 6

Aiyer HS, Kichambare S, Gupta RC 2008. Prevention of oxidative DNA damage by bioactive berry components. Nutritional Cancer. 60

Ajai K. Chemical composition of the essential oil from fresh leaves of Melaleuca leucadendron L. from north India. Journal of Essential Oil-Bearing Plants. CABI Abstracts.

Akatsuka, I. (1990). Introduction to applied phycology. The Hague: SPB Academic Pub. bv.

Akihisa, Toshihiro; Higo, Naoki; Tokuda, Harukuni; Ukiya, Motohiko; Akazawa, Hiroyuki; Tochigi, Yuichi; Kimura, Yumiko; Suzuki, Takashi et al. (2007). "Cucurbitane-type triterpenoids from the fruits of Momordica charantia and their cancer chemopreventive effects". Journal of Natural Products 70

Allaby, M. (1998). A dictionary of plant sciences (2nd ed.). New York: Oxford University Press.

Allahverdiyev, A; Duran, N; Ozguven, M; Koltas, S (2004). "Antiviral activity of the volatile oils of L. Against virus type-2". Phytomedicine 11

Almajano, M. Pilar; Carbó, Rosa; Jiménez, J. Angel López; Gordon, Michael H. (2008). "Antioxidant and antimicrobial activities of tea infusions". Food Chemistry 108

Amer A. Repellency effect of forty-one essential oils against Aedes, American Chemical Society.Biology of Plants 2005

Anderson T, Foght J (2001). "Weight loss and delayed gastric emptying following a South American herbal preparation in overweight patients". J Hum Nutr Diet 14

Anopheles and Culex mosquitoes. Parasitol Res. 2006

American Journal of Botany. (n.d.). from http://www.amjbot.org

American Journal of Clinical Nutrition. (n.d.). Retrieved June 19, 2014, from http://ajcn.nutrition.org/content/by/year

Andrade, G; E Esteban, L Velasco, MJ Lorite, EJ Bedmar (1997). "Isolation and identification of N2-fixing microorganisms from the rhizosphere of Capparis spinosa (L.).". Plant and Soil (Kluwer Academic Publishers) 197

Angier, B. (1978). Field guide to medicinal wild plants. Harrisburg, Pa.: Stackpole Books.

"Antimicrobial activity of Calendula officinalis petal extracts against fungi, as well as Gram-negative and Gram-positive clinical pathogens". Complement Ther Clin Pract 18

Aphrodisiac activity of methanol extract of leaves of Passiflora incarnata Linn. in mice". Phytotherapy Research 17

Appa Rao MVR, Srinivas K, Koteshwar Rao T. "The effect of Mandookaparni (Centella asiatica) on the general mental ability (medhya) of mentally retarded children". J. Res Indian Med. 1973

Arrigoni-Blank Mde F , Oliveira RL , Mendes SS , et al. Seed germination, phenology, and antiedematogenic activity of Peperomia pellucida (L.) H. B. K. BMC Pharmacol . 2002

Aronson, J. (2009). Meyler's side effects of herbal medicines. Amsterdam: Elsevier. Auf'mkolk, M.; Ingbar, J. C.; Kubota, K.; Amir, S. M.; Ingbar, S. H. (1985). "Extracts and Auto-Oxidized Constituents of Certain Plants Inhibit the Receptor-Binding and the Biological Activity of Graves' Immunoglobulins". Endocrinology 116

Austin, DF (2004). Florida Ethnobotany. Boca Raton, FL: CRC Press.

Australian journal of herbal medicine. (n.d.). Concord West, N.S.W.: National Herbalists Association of Australia.

Avadhani, Mythili et al.; The Sweetness and Bitterness of Sweet Flag [Acorus calamus L.] – A Review; Research Journal of Pharmaceutical, Biological and Chemical Sciences, Volume 4, Issue 2

Awad, Rosalie; Muhammad, Asim; Durst, Tony; Trudeau, Vance L.; Arnason, John T. (2009). "Bioassay-guided fractionation of lemon balm (Melissa officinalisL.) using anin vitromeasure of GABA transaminase activity". Phytotherapy Research 23

Aziba PI , Adedeji A , Ekor M , Adeyemi O (2001). "Analgesic activity of Peperomia pellucida aerial parts in mice". Fitoterapia 72

Babykutty, S.; Padikkala, J.; Sathiadevan, P. P.; Vijayakurup, V.; Azis, T. K.; Srinivas, P.; Gopala, S. (2008). "Apoptosis induction of Centella asiatica on human breast cancer cells". African journal of traditional, complementary, and alternative medicines : AJTCAM / African Networks on Ethnomedicines 6

Badar, VA; Thawani, VR; Wakode, PT; Shrivastava, MP; Gharpure, KJ; Hingorani, LL; Khiyani, RM (2005). "Efficacy of Tinospora cordifolia in allergic rhinitis". Journal of Ethnopharmacology 96

Bailey DG, Dresser GK (2004). "Interactions between grapefruit juice and cardiovascular drugs". Am J Cardiovasc Drugs

Bailey, L.H.; Bailey, E.Z.; the staff of the Liberty Hyde Bailey Hortorium. 1976. Hortus third: A concise dictionary of plants cultivated in the United States and Canada. Macmillan, New York.

Balakumbahan, R.; K. Rajamani and K. Kumanan (29 December 2010). Acorus calamus. Journal of Medicinal Plants Research 4 (25): 2740–2745. Retrieved 14 May 2011.

Barnard, Edward S. & Yates, Sharon Fass, ed. (1998). "Trees". Reader's Digest North American Wildlife: Trees and Nonflowering Plants. The Reader's Digest Association, Inc.

Barnes, J., & Anderson, L. (2002). Herbal medicines: A guide for healthcare professionals. (2nd ed.). London: Pharmaceutical Press.

Bakshi N., Kumar P., Sharma M. "Antidermatophytic activity of some alkaloids from Solanum dulcamara." Indian Drugs. 45

Barton, DL; Soori, GS; Bauer, BA; Sloan, JA; Johnson, PA; Figueras, C; Duane, S; Mattar, B et al. (2010). "Pilot study of Panax quinquefolius (American ginseng) to improve cancer-related fatigue: a randomized, double-blind, dose-finding evaluation: NCCTG trial N03CA.". Supportive care in cancer : official journal of the Multinational Association of Supportive Care in Cancer 18

Bastos JF. Moreira IJ. Ribeiro TP. Medeiros IA. Antoniolli AR. De Sousa DP. Santos MR. Hypotensive and vasorelaxant effects of citronellol, a monoterpene alcohol, in rats. Basic & Clinical Pharmacology & Toxicology. 106. 2010

Bayma JD , Arruda MS , Müller AH , Arruda AC , Canto WC . A dimeric ArC 2 compound from Peperomia pellucida . Phytochemistry . 2000

Beal, J. (1981). Natural products as medicinal agents: Plenary lectures of the International Research Congress on Medicinal Plant Research, Strasbourg, July 1980. Stuttgart: Hippokrates Verlag.

Bean, W. J. (1970). Trees and Shrubs Hardy in the British Isles. John Murray, London.

Beloin, N.; Gbeassor, M.; Akpagana, K.; Hudson, J.; De Soussa, K.; Koumaglo, K.; Arnason, J. T. (2005). "Ethnomedicinal uses of Momordica charantia (Cucurbitaceae) in Togo and relation to its phytochemistry and biological activity". Journal of Ethnopharmacology 96

Benedek B., Geisz N., Jäger W., Thalhammer T., Kopp B. Choleretic effects of yarrow (Achillea millefolium s.l.) in the isolated perfused rat liver. Phytomedicine 2006

Benedek, Birgit; Kopp, Brigitte (2007). "Achillea millefolium L. S.l. Revisited: Recent findings confirm the traditional use". Wiener Medizinische Wochenschrift 157

Bensky. Clavey. Stoger. (2004). Gamble Chinese Herbal Medicine

Bensky, Dan; Andrew Gamble, Steven Clavey, Erich Stöger (2004). Chinese Herbal Medicine: Materia Medica, 3rd Edition. Eastland Press.

Bent S, Kane C, Shinohara K, et al (February 2006). "Saw palmetto for benign prostatic hyperplasia". N. Engl. J. Med. 354

Blevi, V., & Sween, G. (1993). Aromatherapy. New York: Avon Books.

Balchin, M. (2006). Aromatherapy Science: A guide for healthcare professionals. London [u.a.: Pharmaceutical Press.

Bhatnagar M. Sisodia SS. Antisecretory and antiulcer activity of Asparagus racemosus Willd. against indomethacin plus phyloric ligation-induced gastric ulcer in rats. Journal of Herbal Pharmacotherapy. 6

Bialonska D, Kasimsetty SG, Khan SI, Ferreira D (11 November 2009). "Urolithins, intestinal microbial metabolites of Pomegranate ellagitannins, exhibit potent antioxidant activity in a cell-based assay". J Agric Food Chem 57

Bilušić Vundać V., Brantner A.H., Plazibat M. "Content of polyphenolic constituents and antioxidant activity of some Stachys taxa" Food Chemistry 2007 104

Blamey, M. & Grey-Wilson, C. (1989). Flora of Britain and Northern Europe. Hodder & Stoughton.

Blanco MM, Costa CA, Freire AO, Santos JG, Costa M (March 2009). "Neurobehavioral effect of essential oil of Cymbopogon citratus in mice". Phytomedicine

Bloomfield, H. (1998). Healing anxiety with herbs. New York, NY: HarperCollins.

Blumenthal, M. (2000). Herbal medicine: Expanded Commission E monographs ; herb monographs, based on those created by a Special Expert Committee of the German Federal Institute for Drugs and Medical Devices (1.st ed.). Newton, Mass.: Integrative Medicine Communications.

Boaz M, Leibovitz E, Bar Dayan Y, Wainstein J (2011). "Functional foods in the treatment of type 2 diabetes: olive leaf extract, turmeric and fenugreek, a qualitative review". Func Foods Health Dis 1

Bojo AC , Albano-Garcia E , Pocsidio GN (1994). "The antibacterial activity of Peperomia pellucida (L.) HBK (Piperaceae)". Asia Life Sci 3: 35–44.

^ Ragasa CY , Dumato M , Rideout JA (1998). "Antifungal compounds from Peperomia pellucida". ACGC Chem Res Commun 7

Bopana N. Saxena S. Asparagus racemosus--ethnopharmacological evaluation and conservation needs. [Review] [77 refs] Journal of Ethnopharmacology. 110

Böttger, Stefan; Melzig, Matthias F. (2011). "Triterpenoid saponins of the Caryophyllaceae and Illecebraceae family". Phytochemistry Letters 4

Boyer, Jeanelle; Liu, RH; Rui Hai Liu (May 2004). "Apple phytochemicals and their health benefits". Nutrition journal Cornell University, Ithaca, New York 14853-7201 USA: Department of Food Science and Institute of Comparative and Environmental Toxicology 3

Boyle, P; Robertson C, Lowe F, Roehrborn C (Apr 2004). "Updated meta-analysis of clinical trials of Serenoa repens extract in the treatment of symptomatic benign prostatic hyperplasia". BJU Int 93

Bradley (1992). British Herbal Compendium 1. Bournemouth, England: British Herbal Medicine Association.

Bradwejn, J.; Zhou, Y.; Koszycki, D.; Shlik, J. (2000). "A double-blind, placebo-controlled study on the effects of Gotu Kola (Centella asiatica) on acoustic startle response in healthy subjects". Journal of clinical psychopharmacology 20

Bramati, Lorenzo; Minoggio, Markus; Gardana, Claudio; Simonetti, Paolo; Mauri, Pierluigi; Pietta, Piergiorgio (2002). "Quantitative Characterization of Flavonoid Compounds in Rooibos Tea (Aspalathus linearis) by LC−UV/DAD". Journal of Agricultural and Food Chemistry 50

Braun, L., & Cohen, M. (2006). Herbs and Natural Supplements Inkling an Evidence-Based Guide. London: Elsevier Health Sciences APAC.

Bremness, L. (1988). The complete book of herbs. New York: Viking Studio Books.

Bressler R (2006). "Grapefruit juice and drug interactions. Exploring mechanisms of this interaction and potential toxicity for certain drugs". Geriatrics 61

Brickell, C. (1994). The Royal Horticultural Society gardeners' encyclopedia of plants and flowers (Rev. ed.). London: Dorling Kindersley.

Brinkhause, B., Lindner, M., et al., "Chemical, Pharmacological and Clinical Profile of The East Asian Medical Plant 2000

British pharmacopoeia 1975. (1975). London: H.M.S.O.

British pharmacopoeia 2013. (2013). London: H.M.S.O.

Brown, D. (1996). Aromatherapy. Lincolnwood, Ill.: NTC Pub.

Brunke, E. (1986). Progress in essential oil research: Proceedings of the International Symposium on Essential Oils, Holzminden/Neuhaus, Federal Republic of Germany, September 18-21, 1985. Berlin: W. de Gruyter.

Bui LT, Nguyen DT, Ambrose PJ (2006). "Blood pressure and heart rate effects following a single dose of bitter orange". The Annals of Pharmacotherapy 40

Burdette JE, Liu J, Chen SN, Fabricant DS, Piersen CE, Barker EL, Pezzuto JM, Mesecar A, Van Breemen RB, Farnsworth NR, Bolton JL (2003). "Black cohosh acts as a mixed competitive ligand and partial agonist of the serotonin receptor". J. Agric. Food Chem. 51

Burk D.R., Cichacz Z.A., Daskalova S.M. Aqueous extract of Achillea millefolium L. (Asteraceae) inflorescences suppresses lipopolysaccharide-induced inflammatory responses in RAW 264.7 murine macrophages. Journal of Medicinal Plant Research 2010

Caceres, A. "Plants used in Guatemala for the treatment of gastrointestinal disorders. 1. Screening of 84 plants against enterobacteria." J. Ethnopharmacol. 1990

Canning S, Waterman M, Orsi N, Ayres J, Simpson N, Dye L (March 2010). "The efficacy of Hypericum perforatum (St John's wort) for the treatment of premenstrual syndrome: a randomized, double-blind, placebo-controlled trial". CNS Drugs 24

Carson, C. F.; Hammer, K. A.; Riley, T. V. (2006). "Melaleuca alternifolia (Tea Tree) Oil: a Review of Antimicrobial and Other Medicinal Properties". Clinical Microbiology Reviews 19

Cassileth, B. (1998). The alternative medicine handbook: The complete reference guide to alternative and complementary therapies. New York: W.W. Norton.

Castleman, M., & Hendler, S. (1991). The healing herbs: The ultimate guide to the curative power of nature's medicines. Emmaus, Pa.: Rodale Press.

Castner, J., & Timme, S. (1998). A field guide to medicinal and useful plants of the Upper Amazon. Gainesville, FL: Feline Press.

Castro, M. (1991). The complete homeopathy handbook: A guide to everyday health care. New York: St. Martin's Press.

Cataldo, A., Gasbarro, V., et al., "Effectiveness of the Combination of Alpha Tocopherol, Rutin, Melilotus, and Centella asiatica in The Treatment of Patients With Chronic Venous Insufficiency", Minerva Cardioangiology, 2001

Ceccarelli N., Curadi M., Picciarelli P., Martelloni L., Sbrana C., Giovannetti M. "Globe artichoke as a functional food" Mediterranean Journal of Nutrition and Metabolism 2010

Cecchini C, Cresci A, Coman MM, et al. (June 2007). "Antimicrobial activity of seven hypericum entities from central Italy". Planta Med. 73

Cerda JJ, Robbins FL, Burgin CW, Baumgartner TG, Rice RW (September 1988). "The effects of grapefruit pectin on patients at risk for coronary heart disease without altering diet or lifestyle". Clin Cardiol 11

Chaiyana W., Okonogi S."Inhibition of cholinesterase by essential oil from food plant". Phytomedicine. 2012.

Chan A, Graves V, Shea TB, A For prevention of dementia: (2006). Journal of Alzheimer's Disease 9

Chan E (1993). "Displacement of bilirubin from albumin by berberine". Biology of the Neonate 63

Chan, E.W.C. et al. (2009). "Effects of different drying methods on the antioxidant properties of leaves and tea of ginger species". Food Chemistry 113

Chan Y.-S., Cheng L.-N., Wu J.-H., Chan E., Kwan Y.-W., Lee S.M.-Y., Leung G.P.-H., Yu P.H.-F., Chan S.-W.,"A review of the pharmacological effects of Arctium lappa (burdock)" [Article in Press] Inflammopharmacology 2010

Chen, G, Sun, W-B, & Sun, H. (2007). Ploidy variation in Buddleja L. (Buddlejaceae) in the Sino - Himalayan region and its biogeographical implications. Botanical Journal of the Linnean Society. 2007

Chen R., Liu Z., Zhao J., Chen R., Meng F., Zhang M., Ge W. "Antioxidant and immunobiological activity of water-soluble polysaccharide fractions purified from Acanthopanax senticosu" Food Chemistry 2011

Chevallier, A. (1996). The encyclopedia of medicinal plants. New York: DK Pub.

Chevallier, A. (2000). Natural health encyclopedia of herbal medicine (2nd American ed.). New York: DK Pub.

Cheung SC, Szeto YT, Benzie IF (March 2007). "Antioxidant protection of edible oils". Plant Foods Hum Nutr 62

Chiang, Y. M.; Lo, C. P.; Chen, Y. P.; Wang, S. Y.; Yang, N. S.; Kuo, Y. H.; Shyur, L. F. (2005). "Ethyl caffeate suppresses NF-κB activation and its downstream inflammatory mediators, iNOS, COX-2, and PGE2in vitroor in mouse skin". British Journal of Pharmacology 146

Chidrawar, VR; Patel, KN; Sheth, NR; Shiromwar, SS; Trivedi, P (2011). "Antiobesity effect of Stellaria media against drug induced obesity in Swiss albino mice". Ayu 32

Chiej, R. (1984). The Macdonald encyclopedia of medicinal plants. London: Macdonald.

Chinese Materia Medica (1998). Beijing University of Traditional Chinese Medicine

Chittenden, F. (1951) RHS Dictionary of Plants plus Supplement. Oxford University Press.

Chopra, R. (1956). Glossary of Indian medicinal plants,. New Delhi: Council of Scientific & Industrial Research.

Chopra, R., & Chopra, R. (1969). Supplement to glossary of Indian medicinal plants. New Delhi: Publications and Information Directorate.

Chopra, R. (1992). Second supplement to Glossary of Indian medicinal plants with active principles. New Delhi: Publications & Information Directorate, CSIR.

Chopra, R. N.; Nayar, S. L.; Chopra, I. C. Glossary of Indian Medicinal Plants. 1986. New Delhi: Council of Scientific and Industrial Research.

Choudhary M.I., Jalil S., Todorova M., Trendafilova A., Mikhova B., Duddeck H. Inhibitory effect of lactone fractions and individual components from three species of the Achillea millefolium complex of Bulgarian origin on the human neutrophils respiratory burst activity. Natural Product Research 2007

Chui C.H., Gambari R., Lau F.Y., Teo I.T.N., Ho K.P., Cheng G.Y.M., Ke B., Higa T., Kok H.L., Chan A.S.C., Tang J.C.O."Anti-cancer potential of traditional Chinese herbal medicines and microbial fermentation products." Minerva Biotecnologica. 17. 2005.

Clarke, D. L. (1988). W. J. Bean Trees and Shrubs Hardy in the British Isles, Supplement. John Murray

Clement, Charles R.; de Cristo-Araújo, Michelly; d'Eeckenbrugge, Geo Coppens; Alves Pereira, Alessandro; Picanço-Rodrigues, Doriane (6 January 2010). "Origin and Domestication of Native Amazonian Crops". Diversity 2

Compendium of medicinal plants. (2004). Delhi, India: National Institute of Industrial Research.

Commission E monographs. (1998). American Botanical Council.

Committee on Comparative Toxicity of Naturally Occurring Carcinogens, Board on Environmental Studies and Toxicology, Commission on Life Sciences, and National Research Council (1996). Carcinogens and anticarcinogens in the human diet: a comparison of naturally occurring and synthetic substances. National Academy Press, Washington, D.C.

Conti B., Canale A., Bertoli A., Gozzini F., Pistelli L. Essential oil composition and larvicidal activity of six

Mediterranean aromatic plants against the mosquito Aedes albopictus (Diptera: Culicidae). Parasitology Research 2010

Coombes, A. (1985). Dictionary of plant names. Portland, Or.: Timber Press.

Coon JT, Ernst E. Andrographis paniculata: a systematic review of safety and efficacy, Planta, 2004

Coon, N. (1977). The dictionary of useful plants. Emmaus: Roodale Press.

Culpepers British Herbal - Pub. William Nicholson and Son - C. 1905 (re-print of the 1653 original)

Cummings, D., & Holmes, A. (n.d.). The medicinal gardening handbook: A complete guide to growing, harvesting, and using healing herbs.

Dasanayake, Ananda P.; Silverman, Amanda J.; Warnakulasuriya, Saman (2010). "Maté drinking and oral and oro-pharyngeal cancer: A systematic review and meta-analysis". Oral Oncology 46

Davidson, A. (1999). The Oxford companion to food. Oxford: Oxford University Press.

Davis & Company Parke (1909). Manual of therapeutics. Parke, Davis & Co.

Davydov M, Krikorian AD. (October 2000). "Eleutherococcus senticosus (Rupr. & Maxim.) Maxim. (Araliaceae) as an adaptogen: a closer look". Journal of Ethnopharmacology 72

de Mesquita, M., et al. "Cytotoxic activity of Brazilian Cerrado plants used in traditional medicine against cancer cell lines." J Ethnopharmacol. 2009

de Lourdes Arruzazabala, M.; Molina, V.; Más, R.; Carbajal, D.; Marrero, D.; González, V.; Rodríguez, E. (2007). "Effects of coconut oil on testosterone-induced prostatic hyperplasia in Sprague-Dawley rats". Journal of Pharmacy and Pharmacology 59

Dedhia RC, McVary KT (June 2008). "Phytotherapy for lower urinary tract symptoms secondary to benign prostatic hyperplasia". J. Urol. 179 (6): 2119–2125.

Dekosky, S. T.; Williamson, J. D.; Fitzpatrick, A. L.; Kronmal, R. A.; Ives, D. G.; Saxton, J. A.; Lopez, O. L.; Burke, G. et al. (2008). "Ginkgo biloba for Prevention of Dementia: A Randomized Controlled Trial". Journal of the American Medical Association 300

Devi, P. U.; Ganasoundari, A. (March 1999). "Modulation of glutathione and antioxidant enzymes by Ocimum sanctum and its role in protection against radiation injury". Indian Journal of Experimental Biology 37

Dew, Tristan P.; Day, Andrea J.; Morgan, Michael R. A. (2005). "Xanthine Oxidase Activity in Vitro: Effects of Food

Extracts and Components". Journal of Agricultural and Food Chemistry 53

Dhama, K., & Dhama, S. (1994). Homoeopathy: The complete handbook. New Delhi: UBS ' Distributors. Complete Homeopathy Handbook 1996 Castro Dictionary catalog of the National Agricultural Library, 1862-1965. (1967). New York: Rowman and Littlefield.

Djavan B, Fong YK, Chaudry A, et al. (2005). "Progression delay in men with mild symptoms of bladder outlet obstruction: a comparative study of phytotherapy and watchful waiting". World J Urol 23 (4): 253–6.

Dos, Santos-Neto, Ll; De, Vilhena, Toledo, Ma; Medeiros-Souza, P; De, Souza, Ga (December 2006). "The use of herbal medicine in Alzheimer's disease-a systematic review" (Free full text). Evidence-based complementary and alternative medicine : eCAM 3

Drugs and Supplements. (n.d.). Retrieved from http://www.mayoclinic.org/drugs-supplements

Duke, J. (1992). Handbook of edible weeds. Boca Raton: CRC Press.

Duke, J. (2000). The green pharmacy herbal handbook: Your comprehensive reference to the best herbs for healing. Emmaus, Pa.: Rodale Reach

Duke. J. A. and Ayensu. E. S. Medicinal Plants of China. Reference Publications, Inc. 1985

Dumitru, Alina F.; Shamji, Mohamed; Wagenmann, Martin; Hindersin, Simone; Scheckenbach, Kathrin; Greve, Jens; Klenzner, Thomas; Hess, Lorenzo et al. (2011). "Petasol butenoate complex (Ze 339) relieves allergic rhinitis–induced nasal obstruction more effectively than desloratadine". Journal of Allergy and Clinical Immunology 127

Ebadi, M. (2002). Pharmacodynamic basis of herbal medicine. Boca Raton, Fla.: CRC Press.

Ebadi, M., & Ebadi, M. (2008). Desk reference of clinical pharmacology (2nd ed.). Boca Raton: CRC Press.

Ebrahimi, Sedigheh; Soheil Ashkani Esfahani, Azizollah Poormahmudi. (2011). "Investigating the efficacy of Zizyphus jujuba on neonatal jaundice". Iranian Journal of Pediatrics 21

Edes, R. (1883). Therapeutic handbook of the United States pharmacopoeia: Being a condensed statement of the physiological and toxic action, medicinal value, methods of administration and doses of the drugs and preparations in the latest edition of the U.S. pharmacopoeia ... New York: William Wood and.

El Bardai S, Lyoussi B, Wibo M, Morel N (May 2001). "Pharmacological evidence of hypotensive activity of Marrubium vulgare and Foeniculum vulgare in spontaneously hypertensive rat". Clin. Exp. Hypertens. 23

Elsabagh, Sarah; Hartley, David E.; Ali, Osama; Williamson, Elizabeth M.; File, Sandra E. (2005). "Differential cognitive effects of Ginkgo biloba after acute and chronic treatment in healthy young volunteers". Psychopharmacology 179

Erichsen-Brown, Charlotte (1989). Medicinal and Other Uses of North American Plants: A Historical Survey with Special Reference to the Eastern Indian Tribes. Dover Publications

Erika Svangård, Ulf Göransson, Zozan Hocaoglu, Joachim Gullbo, Rolf Larsson,, Per Claeson and Lars Bohlin, 2004. "Cytotoxic Cyclotides from Viola tricolor" Journal of Natural Products 67

Estrogen-like activity of ginsenoside Rg1 derived from Panax notoginseng". The Journal of Clinical Endocrinology and Metabolism 87

Ettefagh K.A., Burns J.T., Junio H.A., Kaatz G.W., Cech N.B., "Goldenseal (Hydrastis canadensis L.) Extracts Synergistically Enhance the Antibacterial Activity of Berberine via Efflux Pump Inhibition", Planta Medica 2010

Evans, P. (1961). A modern herbal. San Francisco: Porpoise Bookshop.

A Modern Herbal 1931 Grieve

Ewing, G. (1971). Topics in chemical instrumentation; a volume of reprints from the Journal of chemical education. Easton, Pa.: Chemical Education Pub.

Facciola, S. (1998). Cornucopia II: A source book of edible plants. Vista, CA: Kampong Publications.

Farag RS. Chemical and biological evaluation of the essential oils of different Melaleuca species. Phytother Res. Jan2004;18(1):30-35.

Lee CK. A new norlupene from the leaves of Melaleuca leucadendron. J Nat Prod.

Farnsworth, N. R.; Draus, F. J.; Sager, R. W.; Bianculli, J. A. (2006). "Studies on Vinca major L. (Apocynaceae) I. Isolation of perivincine". Journal of the American Pharmaceutical Association 49

Fehske, Christian J.; Leuner, Kristina; Müller, Walter E. (2009). "Ginkgo biloba extract (EGb761®) influences monoaminergic neurotransmission via inhibition of NE uptake, but not MAO activity after chronic treatment". Pharmacological Research 60

Fern, K. Plants for a Future: Edible and Useful Plants for a Healthier World.

Hampshire: Permanent Publications, 1997.

Fernández S, Wasowski C, Paladini AC, Marder M (2004). "Sedative and sleep-enhancing properties of linarin, a flavonoid-isolated from Valeriana officinalis". Pharmacol Biochem Behav 77

Figueirinha A. Cruz MT. Francisco V. Lopes MC. Batista MT. Anti-inflammatory activity of Cymbopogon citratus leaf infusion in lipopolysaccharide-stimulated dendritic cells: contribution of the polyphenols. Journal of Medicinal Food. 13

Figueroa A, Sanchez-Gonzalez MA, Wong A, Arjmandi BH (2012). "Watermelon extract supplementation reduces ankle blood pressure and carotid augmentation index in obese adults with prehypertension or hypertension". American journal of hypertension 25

Filip, Rosana; Lotito, Silvina B.; Ferraro, Graciela; Fraga, Cesar G. (2000). "Antioxidant activity of Ilex paraguariensis and related species". Nutrition Research 20

Foster, S., & Duke, J. (1990). A field guide to medicinal plants: Eastern and central North America. Boston: Houghton Mifflin.

Francois, G., et al. "Antimalarial and cytotoxic potential of four quassinoids from Hannoa chlorantha and Hannoa klaineana, and their structure-activity relationships." Int. J. Parasitol. 1998

Fu, P.P., Yang, Y.C., Xia, Q., Chou, M.C., Cui, Y.Y., Lin G., "Pyrrolizidine alkaloids-tumorigenic components in Chinese herbal medicines and dietary supplements", Journal of Food and Drug Analysis, Vol. 10, No. 4, 2002

Fugh-Berman, Adriane (2000). "Herb-drug interactions". The Lancet 355

Furst, Peter T. (1976). Hallucinogens and Culture. Chandler & Sharp.

Gadang, V; Gilbert, W; Hettiararchchy, N; Horax, R; Katwa, L; Devareddy, L (2011). "Dietary bitter melon seed increases peroxisome proliferator-activated receptor-γ gene expression in adipose tissue, down-regulates the nuclear factor-κB expression, and alleviates the symptoms associated with metabolic syndrome". Journal of medicinal food 14

Gadow, A.Von; Joubert, E.; Hansmann, C.F. (1997). "Comparison of the antioxidant activity of rooibos tea (Aspalathus linearis) with green, oolong and black tea". Food Chemistry 60

Gaginella, T. (1997). Biochemical pharmacology as an approach to gastrointestinal disorders: Basic science to clinical perspectives (1996) : IUPHAR GI Pharmacology Symposium. Dordrecht: Kluwer Academic.

Ganzera M, Aberham A, Stuppner H (May 2006). "Development and validation of an HPLC/UV/MS method for simultaneous determination of 18 preservatives in grapefruit seed extract". J. Agric. Food Chem. 54

Gautam M. Saha S. Bani S. Kaul A. Mishra S. Patil D. Satti NK. Suri KA. Gairola S. Suresh K. Jadhav S. Qazi GN. Patwardhan B. Immunomodulatory activity of Asparagus racemosus on systemic Th1/Th2 immunity: implications for immunoadjuvant potential. Journal of Ethnopharmacology. 121

Grae, I. (1974). Nature's colors; dyes from plants. New York: Macmillan.

Gray, A., & Sullivant, W. (1848). A manual of the botany of the northern United States from New England to Wisconsin and south to Ohio and Pennsylvania inclusive: (the mosses and liverworts by Wm. S. Sullivant,) arranged according to the natural system. Boston: J. Munroe.

Geller SE, Shulman LP, van Breemen RB, et al. (2009). "Safety and efficacy of black cohosh and red clover for the management of vasomotor symptoms: a randomized controlled trial". Menopause (New York, N.Y.) 16

Genders. R. Scented Flora of the World. Robert Hale. London. 1994

Gentry EJ, Jampani HB, Keshavarz-Shokri A, et al. (October 1998). "Antitubercular natural products: berberine from the roots of commercial Hydrastis canadensis powder. Isolation of inactive 8-oxotetrahydrothalifendine, canadine, beta-hydrastine, and two new quinic acid esters, hycandinic acid esters-1 and -2". Journal of Natural Products 61

Germplasm Resources Information Network. United States Department of Agriculture. 1997-05-22. Retrieved 2010-04-12.

Ghalayini IF, Al-Ghazo MA, Harfeil MN 2011. Prophylaxis and therapeutic effects of raspberry (Rubus idaeus) on renal stone formation in Balb/c mice. Int Braz J Urol. 37

Ghosh, P. C., et al. "Antitumor plants. IV. Constituents of Simarouba versicolor." Lloydia. 1977

Ghosh S, Sharma AK, Kumar S, Tiwari SS, Rastogi S, Srivastava S, Singh M, Kumar R, Paul S, Ray DD, Rawat AK "In vitro and in vivo efficacy of Acorus calamus extract against Rhipicephalus (Boophilus) microplus." Parasitol Res. 2011

Gião MS, Pestana D, Faria A, Guimarães JT, Pintado ME, Calhau C, Azevedo I, Malcata FX., 2010. Effects of extracts of selected medicinal plants upon hepatic oxidative stress. Journal Medicinal Food. 13

Gibbs A, Green C, Doctor VM. (1983). "Isolation and anticoagulant properties of polysaccharides of Typha Augustata and Daemonorops species". Thromb Res. 32

Gilani A.H., Bashir S., Khan A.-u."Pharmacological basis for the use of Borago officinalis in gastrointestinal, respiratory and cardiovascular disorders". Journal of Ethnopharmacology. 114

Giles M., Ulbricht C., Khalsa K.P.S., DeFranco Kirkwood C., Park C., Basch E., "Butterbur: An evidence-based systematic review by the natural standard research collaboration Journal of Herbal Pharmacotherapy 2005

God J, Tate PL, Larcom LL 2010. Red raspberries have antioxidant effects that play a minor role in the killing of stomach and colon cancer cells. Nutritional Research. 30

Godevac D, Tesević V, Vajs V, Milosavljević S, Stanković M., 2009. Antioxidant properties of raspberry seed extracts on micronucleus distribution in peripheral blood lymphocytes. Food Chem 47

Godowski, KC (1989). "Antimicrobial action of sanguinarine". The Journal of clinical dentistry 1

Golshahi H., Ghasemi E., Mehranzade E. (2011). "Antibacterial activity of Ocimum sanctum extract against E. coli, S. aureus and P. aeruginosa". Clinical Biochemistry. Conference: 12th Iranian Congress of Biochemistry, ICB and 4th International Congress of Biochemistry and Molecular Biology 44

Goodner, K.L. et al.; Mahattanatawee, K; Plotto, A; Sotomayor, J; Jordan, M (2006). "Aromatic profiles of Thymus hyemalis and Spanish T. vulgaris essential oils by GC–MS/GC–O". Industrial Crops and Products 24

Gregory PJ, Sperry M, Wilson AF (January 2008). "Dietary supplements for osteoarthritis". Am Fam Physician 77

Grieve, M. (1971). A modern herbal; the medicinal, culinary, cosmetic and economic properties, cultivation and folk-lore of herbs, grasses, fungi, shrubs, & trees with all their modern scientific uses,. New York: Dover Publications.

Griffith, J.Q.; J.F. Couch, M. A. Lindauer (1944). "Effect of Rutin on Increased Capillary Fragility". Proc Soc Exp Biol Med March 55

Grover, J. K.; Yadav, S. P. (2004). "Pharmacological actions and potential uses of Momordica charantia: A review". Journal of Ethnopharmacology 93

Grubben, G.J.H. & Denton, O.A. (2004) Plant Resources of Tropical Africa 2. Vegetables. PROTA Foundation, Wageningen; Backhuys, Leiden; CTA, Wageningen

Grujic-Jovanovic S., Skaltsa H.D., Marin P., Sokovic M. "Composition and antibacterial activity of the essential oil of six Stachys species from Serbia" Flavour and Fragrance Journal 2004 19

Gualtiero Simonetti (1990). Stanley Schuler, ed. Simon & Schuster's Guide to Herbs and Spices. Simon & Schuster, Inc.

Gualtiero Simonetti (1990). Stanley Schuler, ed. Simon & Schuster's Guide to Herbs and Spices. Simon & Schuster, Inc.

Guenther, E. (1949). The essential oils. New York: D. Van Nostrand.

Guo LY. Hung TM. Bae KH. Shin EM. Zhou HY. Hong YN. Kang SS. Kim HP. Kim YS.,"Anti-inflammatory effects of schisandrin isolated from the fruit of Schisandra chinensis Baill." European Journal of Pharmacology. 591

Guo, R; Pittler, MH; Ernst, E (2007). "Herbal medicines for the treatment of allergic rhinitis: A systematic review". Annals of allergy, asthma & immunology : official publication of the American College of Allergy, Asthma, & Immunology 99

Gurudeeban S.; Satyavani K., Ramanathan T. (2010). "Bitter Apple (Citrullus colocynthis): An Overview of Chemical Composition and Biomedical Potentials". Asian Journal of Plant Sciences 9

H. J. D. Dorman and S. G. Deans (2000). "Antimicrobial agents from plants: antibacterial activity of plant volatile oils". Journal of Applied Microbiology 88

H. Kohno, Y. Yasui, R. Suzuki, M. Hosokawa, K. Miyashita, T. Tanaka (2004), Dietary seed oil rich in conjugated linolenic acid from bitter melon inhibits azoxymethane-induced rat colon carcinogenesis through elevation of colonic PPAR γ expression and alteration of lipid composition. International Journal of Cancer, volume 110

Ha H.H., Park S.Y., Ko W.S., Kim Y. "Gleditsia sinensis thorns inhibit the production of NO through NF-B suppression in LPS-stimulated macrophages. Journal of Ethnopharmacology. 2008. 118

Hage-Sleiman, R; Mroueh, M; Daher, CF (2011). "Pharmacological evaluation of aqueous extract of Althaea officinalis flower grown in Lebanon". Pharmaceutical biology 49

Hager TJ, Howard LR, Liyanage R, Lay JO, Prior RL (February 2008). "Ellagitannin composition of blackberry as determined by HPLC-ESI-MS and MALDI-TOF-MS". Journal of Agricultural and Food Chemistry 56

Halvorsen BL, Carlsen MH, Phillips KM, et al. (July 2006). "Content of redox-active compounds (ie, antioxidants) in foods consumed in the United States". The American Journal of Clinical Nutrition 84

Hamamelitannin from Witch Hazel (Hamamelis virginiana) Displays Specific Cytotoxic Activity against Colon Cancer Cells. Susana Sánchez-Tena, María L. Fernández-Cachón, Anna Carreras, M. Luisa Mateos-Martín, Noelia Costoya, Mary P. Moyer, María J. Nuñez, Josep L. Torres and Marta Cascante, J. Nat. Prod.

Hammer, K; Carson, C; Riley, T; Nielsen, J (2006). "A review of the toxicity of Melaleuca alternifolia (tea tree) oil". Food and Chemical Toxicology 44

Hanelt, Peter; Büttner, R.; Mansfeld, Rudolf; Kilian, Ruth (2001). Mansfeld's Encyclopedia of Agricultural and Horticultural Crops. Springer.

Hannan JM. Marenah L. Ali L. Rokeya B. Flatt PR. Abdel-Wahab YH. Insulin secretory actions of extracts of Asparagus racemosus root in perfused pancreas, isolated islets and clonal pancreatic beta-cells. Journal of Endocrinology. 192

Harborne, J. (1996). Dictionary of plant toxins. Chichester: Wiley.

Harper, Douglas; Online Etymological Dictionary; http://www.etymonline.com/index

Harrison, Lorraine (2012). RHS Latin for gardeners. United Kingdom: Mitchell Beazley.

Haskell CF, Kennedy DO, Wesnes KA, Milne AL, Scholey AB (January 2007). "A double-blind, placebo-controlled, multi-dose evaluation of the acute behavioral effects of guaraná in humans". J. Psychopharmacol. (Oxford) 21

Hartwell, Jonathan L. (1971). Bioactive Plants "Plants used against cancer. A survey". Lloydia

Hausen, B. M. (1993). "Centella asiatica (Indian pennywort), an effective therapeutic but a weak sensitizer". Contact Dermatitis 29 (

Hecht SS, Carmella SG, Murphy SE (1 October 1999). "Effects of watercress consumption on urinary metabolites of nicotine in smokers". Cancer Epidemiol Biomarkers

Heinonen, M (2007). "Antioxidant activity and antimicrobial effect of berry phenolics--a Finnish perspective". Molecular nutrition & food research 51

Heinrich, Clark (2002). Magic Mushrooms in Religion and Alchemy. Rochester: Park Street Press.

Heisy, Rod M. (May 1990). "Allelopathic and Herbicidal Effects of Extracts from Tree of Heaven". American Journal of Botany 77

Henrotin Y, Clutterbuck AL, Allaway D, et al. (February 2010). "Biological actions of curcumin on articular chondrocytes". Osteoarthr. Cartil. 18

Hensel, Andreas; Maas, Mareike; Sendker, Jandirk; Lechtenberg, Matthias; Petereit, Frank; Deters, Alexandra; Schmidt, Thomas & Stark, Timo (2011). "Eupatorium perfoliatum L.: Phytochemistry, traditional use and current applications". Journal of Ethnopharmacology

Herbal therapy, medicinal plants, and natural products: An IPA compilation. (1999). Bethesda, MD: American Society of Health-System Pharmacists.

Herbs and natural supplements: An evidence based guide. (n.d.). Mosby Sydney, Australia.

Hess AM, Sullivan DL (2005). "Potential for toxicity with use of bitter orange extract and guarana for weight loss". The Annals of pharmacotherapy 39

Heywood VH. 1993 "Flowering plants of the world." Oxford University Press, New York

Hillier & Sons. (1977). Hilliers' Manual of Trees and Shrubs, 4th Edition. David & Charles, Newton Abbot, England.

Hirota, N. and Hiroi, M., 1967. 'The later studies on the camphor tree, on the leaf oil of each practical form and its utilisation', Perfumery and Essential Oil Record 58

Hirsch, Pamela; Gladstar, Rosemary (2000). Planting the future: saving our medicinal herbs. Rochester, Vt: Healing Arts Press

Hoa NK, Phan DV, Thuan ND, Ostenson CG (April 2009). "Screening of the hypoglycemic effect of eight Vietnamese herbal drugs". Methods & Findings in Experimental & Clinical Pharmacology 31

Hoffmann, Medical Herbalism: Principles and Practices, Healing Arts Press, 2003

Holliday, P. (1989). A dictionary of plant pathology. Cambridge [England: Cambridge University Press.

Holzl J, Godau P. (1989). "Receptor binding studies with Valeriana officinalis on the benzodiazepine receptor". Planta Medica 55

Hong B; Ji YH; Hong JH; Nam KY; Ahn TY A double-blind crossover study evaluating the efficacy of korean red ginseng in patients with erectile dysfunction: a preliminary report. J Urol. 2002

Huang L.-Z., Huang B.-K., Ye Q., Qin L.-P. "Bioactivity-guided fractionation for anti-fatigue property of Acanthopanax senticosus" Journal of Ethnopharmacology 2011

Huang Yuan, Dong Qi, Qiao Shan-Yi. Studies on the Chemical Constituents From Stellaria media (II). Pharmaceutical Journal of Chinese People's Liberation Army, 2007-03 (abstract) (Article in Chinese)

Hughes, R. Elwyn; Ellery, Peter; Harry, Tim; Jenkins, Vivian; Jones, Eleri (1980). "The dietary potential of the common nettle". Journal of the Science of Food and Agriculture 31

Hunt EJ, Lester CE, Lester EA, Tackett RL. (June 2001). "Effect of St. John's wort on free radical production". Life Sci. 69

Hutchens, A. (1992). A handbook of native American herbs. Boston: [New York]

Huxley, A., ed. (1992). New RHS Dictionary of Gardening. Macmillan

Huyen VT, Phan DV, Thang P, Hoa NK, Ostenson CG (May 2010). "Antidiabetic effect of Gynostemma pentaphyllum tea in randomly assigned type 2 diabetic patients". Hormone & Metabolic Research 42

Iacobellis, N S. et al. (2005). "Antibacterial Activity of Cuminum cyminum L. and Carum carvi L. Essential Oils". Journal of Agricultural and Food Chemistry 53

Index herbariorum. (1990). Bronx, N.Y.: Published and distributed for International Association for Plant Taxonomy by New York Botanical Gardens.

Indian journal of natural products. (1985). Sagar, India: [Indian Society of Pharmacognosy].

ISHS Acta Horticulturae 306: International Symposium on Medicinal and Aromatic Plants, XXIII IHC Isolation and purification of baicalein, wogonin and oroxylin A from the medicinal plant Scutellaria baicalensis by high-speed counter-current chromatography. Hua-Bin Li and Feng Chen, Journal of Chromatography A, 2005, Volume 1074

Ital J Biochem. 1988. Effect of the triterpenoid fraction of Centella asiatica on macromolecules of the connective matrix in human skin fibroblast cultures.

Tenni R, Zanaboni G, De Agostini MP, Rossi A, Bendotti C, Cetta G.

Izzo A.A. Ernst E. (2001). "Interactions Between Herbal Medicines and Prescribed Drugs: A Systematic Review". Drugs (Adis International) 61

J. Östman; M. Britton, eds. (2004), "4.7.3 Alternative Medicine Methods Used to Treat Obesity", Treating and Preventing Obesity: An Evidence Based Review, Wiley-VCH.

Jarald E., Nalwaya N., Sheeja E., Ahmad S., Jamalludin S. (2010). "Comparative study on diuretic activity of few medicinal plants in individual form and in combination form". Indian Drugs 47

Jedlicková Z. Antibacterial properties of the Vietnamese cajeput oil and ocimum oil in combination with antibacterial agents. J Hyg Epidemiol Microbiol Immunol.

Jeong-Kyu KIM, Chang-Soo KANG, Jong-Kwon LEE, Young-Ran KIM, Hye-Yun HAN, Hwa Kyung YUN (2005). "Evaluation of Repellency Effect of Two Natural Aroma Mosquito Repellent Compounds, Citronella and Citronellal". Entomological Research 35

Jiang J.-G., Huang X.-J., Chen J., Lin Q.-S.,"Comparison of the sedative and hypnotic effects of flavonoids, saponins, and polysaccharides extracted from Semen Ziziphus jujube" Natural Produ ct Research 2007 21

Jigna Parekh, Nehal Karathia, Sumitra Chanda (2006). "Screening of some traditionally used medicinal plants for potential antibacterial activity". Indian Journal of Pharmaceutical Sciences 68

Jing, M. et al. (1987). "Study on the mechanism of Valeriana officinalis for infantile viral diarrhea". Yunnan J. Traditional Chin. Med. 8

Jordan P; Wheeler S. (2001). The ultimate mushroom book. Hermes House.

Joseph I. Boullata and Angela M. Nace (2000). "Safety Issues with Herbal Medicine: Common Herbal Medicines". Pharmacotherapy 20

Joubert, E.; Gelderblom, W.C.A.; Louw, A.; De Beer, D. (2008). "South African herbal teas: Aspalathus linearis, Cyclopia spp. And Athrixia phylicoides—A review". Journal of Ethnopharmacology 119

Jung HA, Su BN, Keller WJ, Mehta RG, Kinghorn AD (March 2006). "Antioxidant xanthones from the pericarp of Garcinia mangostana (Mangosteen)". Journal of Agricultural and Food Chemistry 54

Jung S.M., Schumacher H.R., Kim H., Kim M., Lee S.H., Pessler F. "Reduction of urate crystal-induced inflammation by

root extracts from traditional oriental medicinal plants: Elevation of prostaglandin D2levels" Arthritis Research and Therapy 2007 9

Junwei J. Zhu, Christopher A. Dunlap, Robert W. Behle, Dennis R. Berkebile, Brian Wienhold. (2010). Repellency of a wax-based catnip-oil formulation against stable flies. Journal of Agricultural and Food Chemistry, 58

Kade, F.; Miller, W. (1993). "Dose-dependent effects of Ginkgo biloba extraction on cerebral, mental and physical efficiency: a placebo controlled double blind study". British journal of clinical research 4.

Kamal-Eldin A, Moazzami A, Washi S (January 2011). "Sesame seed lignans: potent physiological modulators and possible ingredients in functional foods & nutraceuticals". Recent Pat Food Nutr Agric 3

Kamaldeep Dhawan, Suresh Kumar, Anupam Sharma (2001). "Anti-anxiety studies on extracts of Passiflora incarnata Linneaus [sic]". Journal of Ethnopharmacology 78

Kamaldeep Dhawan & Anupam Sharma (2002). "Antitussive activity of the methanol extract of Passiflora incarnata leaves". Fitoterapia 73

Kamaldeep Dhawan, Suresh Kumar & Anupam Sharma (2003). "Antiasthmatic activity of the methanol extract of leaves of Passiflora incarnata". Phytotherapy Research 17

Kamat JP. Boloor KK. Devasagayam TP. Venkatachalam SR. Antioxidant properties of Asparagus racemosus against damage induced by gamma-radiation in rat liver mitochondria. Journal of Ethnopharmacology. 71

Kamdem D. P., Gage, D. A. (1995). "Chemical Composition of Essential Oil from the Root Bark of Sassafras albidum". Journal of Organic Chemistry 61

Kang IJ, Lee MH (July 2006). "Quantification of para-phenylenediamine and heavy metals in henna dye". Contact Dermatitis 55

Kanwar, Anubha Singh ; Bhutani, Kamlesh Kumar "Effects of Chlorophytum arundinaceum, Asparagus adscendens and Asparagus racemosus on Pro-inflammatory Cytokine and Corticosterone Levels Produced by Stress" . BIOSIS Previews Phytotherapy Research. 24

Kapasakalidis, PG; Rastall, RA; Gordon, MH (2006). "Extraction of polyphenols from processed black currant (Ribes nigrum L.) residues". Journal of Agricultural and Food Chemistry 54

Katsaridis, V.; Papagiannaki C., Aimar E. (2009). "Embolization of brain arteriovenous malformations for cure: because we could and because we should". American Journal of Neuroradiology 30

Katzenschlager, R; Evans, A; Manson, A; Patsalos, PN; Ratnaraj, N; Watt, H; Timmermann, L; Van Der Giessen, R et al. (2004). "Mucuna pruriens in Parkinson's disease: a double blind clinical and pharmacological study". Journal of Neurology, Neurosurgery & Psychiatry 75

Kaufman, PB; Duke, JA; Brielmann, H; Boik, J; Hoyt, JE (1997). "A comparative survey of leguminous plants as sources of the isoflavones, genistein and daidzein: Implications for human nutrition and health". Journal of alternative and complementary medicine 3 Kaunitz, H. (1986). "Medium chain triglycerides (MCT) in aging and arteriosclerosis". Journal of Environmental Pathology, Toxicology and Oncology : official organ of the International Society for Environmental Toxicology and Cancer 6 Kennedy, D. O.; Little, W; Scholey, AB (2004). "Attenuation of Laboratory-Induced Stress in Humans After Acute Administration of Melissa officinalis (Lemon Balm)". Psychosomatic Medicine 66

Khan MR , Omoloso AD . Antibacterial activity of Hygrophila stricta and Peperomia pellucida . Fitoterapia . 2002

Khonkarn R. Okonogi S. Ampasavate C. Anuchapreeda S. Investigation of fruit peel extracts as sources for compounds with antioxidant and antiproliferative activities against human cell lines. Food & Chemical Toxicology. 48

Kilham, C. (2000). Tales from the Medicine Trail: Tracking Down the Health Secrets of Shamans, Herbalists, Mystics, Yogis, and Other Healers. [Emmaus PA]: Rodale Press.

Kim, H.; Song, M-J.; Potter, D. (2005). "Medicinal efficacy of plants utilized as temple food in traditional Korean Buddihsm". Journal of Ethnopharmacology 104

Kim, H. J.; Chang, E. J.; Cho, S. H.; Chung, S. K.; Park, H. D.; Choi, S. W. (2002). "Antioxidative activity of resveratrol and its derivatives isolated from seeds of Paeonia lactiflora". Bioscience, biotechnology, and biochemistry 66

Kim, M. H.; Nugroho, A.; Choi, J.; Park, J. H.; Park, H. J. (2011). "Rhododendrin, an analgesic/anti-inflammatory arylbutanoid glycoside, from the leaves of Rhododendron aureum". Archives of Pharmacal Research 34

Kim SJ. Min HY. Lee EJ. Kim YS. Bae K. Kang SS. Lee SK. 'Growth inhibition and cell cycle arrest in the G0/G1 by schizandrin, a dibenzocyclooctadiene lignan isolated from Schisandra chinensis, on T47D human breast cancer cells." Phytotherapy Research. 24

King, J., & Felter, H. (1898). King's American dispensatory (18th ed.). Cincinnati: Ohio Valley

Klepser TB, Klepser ME (1999). "Unsafe and potentially safe herbal therapies". Am J Health-Syst Pharm 56

Ko HC, Wei BL, Chiou WF. The effect of medicinal plants used in Chinese folk medicine on RANTES, Ethnopharmacol, 2006

Koh, H., & Chua, T. (2009). A guide to medicinal plants an illustrated, scientific and medicinal approach. Singapore: World Scientific Pub.

Kraemer, H. (1910). A text-book of botany and pharmacognosy, intended for the use of students of pharmacy, as a reference book for pharmacists, and as a handbook for food and drug analysts, (4th rev. and enl. ed.). Philadelphia & London: J.B. Lippincott Company.

Krafczyk, Nicole; Woyand, Franziska; Glomb, Marcus A. (2009). "Structure-antioxidant relationship of flavonoids from fermented rooibos". Molecular Nutrition & Food Research 53

Krochmal, A., & Krochmal, C. (1984). A field guide to medicinal plants (Updated Times Books pbk. ed.). New York, N.Y.: Times Books.

Kang IJ, Lee MH (July 2006). "Quantification of para-phenylenediamine and heavy metals in henna dye". Contact Dermatitis 55

Kulkarni AP, Mahal HS, Kapoor S, Aradhya SM (February 21, 2007). "In vitro studies on the binding, antioxidant, and cytotoxic actions of punicalagin". J Agric Food Chem 55

Kumar, S. (1998). A complete clinical handbook for every day practice. New Delhi: Indian Books & Periodicals.

Kumar S., Singh Y. V., & Singh, M. (2005). "Agro-History, Uses, Ecology and Distribution of Henna (Lawsonia inermis L. syn. Alba Lam)". Henna: Cultivation, Improvement, and Trade. Jodhpur: Central Arid Zone Research Institute.

Kunkel SD, Elmore CJ, Bongers KS, Ebert SM, Fox DK, et al. (2012) Ursolic Acid Increases Skeletal Muscle and Brown Fat and Decreases Diet-Induced Obesity, Glucose Intolerance and Fatty Liver Disease. PLoS ONE 7

Kurkin VA, Dubishchev AV, Ezhkov VN, Titova IN, Avdeeva EV (2006). "Antidepressant activity of some phytopharmaceuticals and phenylpropanoids". Pharmaceutical Chemistry Journal 40

L. Kumar P., Sharma B., Bakshi N.,"Biological activity of alkaloids from Solanum dulcamara". Natural Product Research. 23. 2009.

Larrosa M, González-Sarrías A, Yáñez-Gascón MJ, Selma MV, Azorín-Ortuño M, Toti S, Tomás-Barberán F, Dolara P, Espín JC (19 July 2009). "Anti-inflammatory properties of a pomegranate extract and its metabolite urolithin-A in a colitis rat model and the effect of colon inflammation on phenolic metabolism". J Nutr Biochem 21

Lauro, Gabriel J.; Francis, F. Jack (2000). Natural Food Colorants Science and Technology. IFT Basic Symposium Series. New York: Marcel Dekker.

Galindo-Cuspinera, V; Westhoff, DC; Rankin, SA (2003). "Antimicrobial properties of commercial annatto extracts against selected pathogenic, lactic acid, and spoilage microorganisms". Journal of food protection 66

Lawrence, B. M., 1995. 'Progress in essential oils', Perfumer and Flavorist, "Leaf Extract Treatment During the Growth Spurt Period Enhances Hippocampal CA3 Neuronal Dendritic Arborization in Rats". Evid Based Complement Alternat Med: 2006.

Lee do Y. Choo BK. Yoon T. Cheon MS. Lee HW. Lee AY. Kim HK. Anti-inflammatory effects of Asparagus cochinchinensis extract in acute and chronic cutaneous inflammation. Journal of Ethnopharmacology. 121

Lee HJ. Jeong HS. Kim DJ. Noh YH. Yuk DY. Hong JT. Inhibitory effect of citral on NO production by suppression of iNOS expression and NF-kappa B activation in RAW264.7 cells. Archives of Pharmacal Research. 31

Lee IA, Joh EH, Kim DH, "Arctigenin Isolated from the Seeds of Arctium lappa Ameliorates Memory Deficits in Mice." Planta Med. 2011

Lee M.-Y., Shin I.-S., Seo C.-S., Ha H., Shin H.-K."Antiasthmatic effects of Gleditsia sinensis in an ovalbumin-induced murine model of asthma". International Journal of Toxicology. 30. 2011

Lee S.-J., Park K., Ha S.-D., Kim W.-J., Moon S.-K. " Gleditsia sinensis thorn extract inhibits human colon cancer cells: The role of ERK1/2, G2/M-phase cell cycle arrest and p53 expression". Phytotherapy Research. 24

Lee, Seung-Joo et al.; Umano, K; Shibamoto, T; Lee, K (2005). "Identification of volatile components in basil (Ocimum basilicum L.) and thyme leaves (Thymus vulgaris L.) and their antioxidant properties". Food Chemistry 91

Lee, YJ; Jin, YR; Lim, WC; Park, WK; Cho, JY; Jang, S; Lee, SK (2003). "Ginsenoside-Rb1 acts as a weak phytoestrogen in MCF-7 human breast cancer cells". Archives of pharmacal research 26

Leite JR, Seabra Mde L, Maluf E, et al. (July 1986). "Pharmacology of lemongrass (Cymbopogon citratus Stapf). III. Assessment of eventual toxic, hypnotic and anxiolytic effects on humans". J Ethnopharmacol 17

Leos-Rivas C., Verde-Star M.J., Torres L.O., Oranday-Cardenas A., Rivas-Morales C., Barron-Gonzalez M.P., Morales-Vallarta M.R., Cruz-Vega D.E. In vitro amoebicidal activity of borage (Borago officinalis) extract on entamoeba histolytica. Journal of Medicinal Food. 14. 2011.

Lesca, P. (1983). Protective effects of ellagic acid and other plant phenols on benzo[a]pyrene-induced neoplasia in mice.

Lewis K (April 2001). "In search of natural substrates and inhibitors of MDR pumps". Journal of Molecular Microbiology and Biotechnology 3

Lewis, WH and Elvin-Lewis, MPF (2003). Medical botany: plants affecting human health. Hoboken, New Jersey; John Wiley & Sons

Li, C. (1974). Chinese herbal medicine. Washington: U.S. Dept. of Health, Education, and Welfare, Public Health Service, National Institutes of Health.

Li, C. (2003). Chinese herbal medicine. San Diego, Calif.: Book Tree.

Li, Tao; Zhang, Hao (2008), "Identification and Comparative Determination of Rhodionin in Traditional Tibetan Medicinal Plants of Fourteen Rhodiola Species by High-Performance Liquid Chromatography-Photodiode Array Detection and Electrospray Ionization-Mass Spectrometry", Chemical & Pharmaceutical Bulletin 56

Li W.-H., Zhang X.-M., Tian R.-R., Zheng Y.-T., Zhao W.-M., Qiu M.-H.,"A new anti-HIV lupane acid from Gleditsia sinensis Lam.". Journal of Asian Natural Products Research. 9. 2007

Lichtenthäler R, Rodrigues RB, Maia JG, Papagiannopoulos M, Fabricius H, Marx

F (Feb 2005). "Total oxidant scavenging capacities of Euterpe oleracea Mart. (Açaí) fruits". Int J Food Science Nutrition 56

Lim, T. K. (2013). Edible medicinal and non-medicinal plants. Dordrecht: Springer.

Lin JK, Chen YC, et al. "Suppression of protein kinase C and nuclear oncogene expression as possible molecular mechanism of cancer chemoprevention by apigenin and curcumin", J Cell Biochem

Lin RD, Mao YW, Leu SJ, Huang CY, Lee MH.,"The immuno-regulatory effects of Schisandra chinensis and its constituents on human monocytic leukemia cells." Molecules. 2011

Lis-Balchin M., Hart S. and Simpson E. (2001). Buchu (Agathosma betulina and A. crenulata, Rutaceae) essential oils: their pharmacological action on guinea-pig ileum and antimicrobial activity on microorganisms. J Pharm Pharmacol.

Liu W. Huang XF. Qi Q. Dai QS. Yang L. Nie FF. Lu N. Gong DD. Kong LY. Guo QL. Asparanin A induces G(2)/M cell cycle arrest and apoptosis in human hepatocellular carcinoma HepG2 cells. Biochemical & Biophysical Research Communications. 381

Loewenfeld, C., & Back, P. (1980). Britain's wild larder. North Pomfret, Vt.: David & Charles.

Lohakachornpan P. Chemical compositions and antimicrobial activities of essential oil from Melaleuca leucadendron var. minor. Thai J Pharma Sci. 2001

Longe, J. (2005). The Gale encyclopedia of alternative medicine (2nd ed.). Detroit: Thomson Gale.

Loudon, J. (1866). Loudon's encyclopaedia of plants; comprising the specific character, description, culture, history, application in the arts, and every other desirable particular respecting all the plants indigenous to cultivated in, or introduced into Britain. (New impression. ed.). London: Longmans, Green

Lowther, Granville; William Worthington. The Encyclopedia of Practical Horticulture: A Reference System of Commercial Horticulture, Covering the Practical and Scientific Phases of Horticulture, with Special Reference to Fruits and Vegetables.

Lu, G.; Lu G, Edwards CG, Fellman JK, Mattinson DS, Navazio J. (February 2003). "Biosynthetic origin of geosmin in red beets (Beta vulgaris L.).". Journal of Agricultural and Food Chemistry (abstract) (American Chemical Society) 12

Luczak, S; Swiatek, L; Daniewski, M (1989). "Phenolic acids in herbs Lysimachia nummularia L. And L. Vulgaris L". Acta poloniae pharmaceutica 46

Lynas, L. (1972). Medicinal and food plants of the North American Indians: A bibliography. Bronx, N.Y.: Library of New York Botanical Garden.

M. M. Lolitkar and M. R. Rajarama Rao (1962), Note on a Hypoglycaemic Principle Isolated from the fruits of Momordica charantia. Journal of the University of Bombay, volume 29

Mabey, Richard; 'Plants with a Purpose: A guide to the everyday use of wild plants', William Collins, Fontana, Glasgow, 1977

MacGregor FB, Abernethy VE, Dahabra S, Cobden I, Hayes PC (1989). "Hepatotoxicity of herbal remedies". British Medical Journal 299

Mahadevan, S.; Park, Y. (2007). "Multifaceted Therapeutic Benefits of Ginkgo biloba L.: Chemistry, Efficacy, Safety, and Uses". Journal of Food Science 73

Major Apoptosis-Inducing Components of Bitter Gourd". Journal of Agricultural and Food Chemistry 56

Mandal SC. Kumar C K A. Mohana Lakshmi S. Sinha S. Murugesan T. Saha BP. Pal M. Antitussive effect of Asparagus racemosus root against sulfur dioxide-induced cough in mice. Fitoterapia. 71

Manniche, Lisa; An Ancient Egyptian Herbal, pg. 74; American University in Cairo Press; Cairo; 2006

Marc Spehr; Günter Gisselmann, Alexandra Poplawski, Jeffrey A. Riffell, Christian H. Wetzel, Richard K. Zimmer, Hanns Hatt (2003). "Identification of a Testicular Odorant Receptor Mediating Human Sperm Chemotaxis". Science 299 (5615): 2054.

Marnewick, Jeanine L.; Rautenbach, Fanie; Venter, Irma; Neethling, Henry; Blackhurst, Dee M.; Wolmarans, Petro; Macharia, Muiruri (2011). "Effects of rooibos (Aspalathus linearis) on oxidative stress and biochemical parameters in adults at risk for cardiovascular disease". Journal of Ethnopharmacology 133

Marzouk, B.; Haloui E., Akremi N., Aouni M., Marzouk Z., Fenina N. (2012). "Antimicrobial and anticoagulant activities of Citrullus colocynthis Schrad. leaves from Tunisia (Medenine)". African Journal of Pharmacy and Pharmacology 6

Matlwaska (2002). "Flavonoid compounds in the flowers of Abutilon

179

indicum (Linn.) Sweet". Acia Poloniac Pharmaceutic - Drug Research 59

Matsumoto T., Hosono-Nishiyama K., Yamada H. , "Antiproliferative and apoptotic effects of butyrolactone lignans from Arctium lappa on leukemic cells" Planta Medica 2006

May, G., et al. "Antiviral activity of aqueous extracts from medicinal plants in tissue cultures." Arzneim-Forsch 1978

Mazza, M.; Capuano, A.; Bria, P.; Mazza, S. (2006). "Ginkgo biloba and donepezil: a comparison in the treatment of Alzheimer's dementia in a randomized placebo-controlled double-blind study". European Journal of Neurology 13

McCabe, Melvina; Gohdes, Dorothy; Morgan, Frank; Eakin, Joanne; Sanders, Margaret; Schmitt, Cheryl (2005). "Herbal Therapies and Diabetes Among Navajo Indians". Diabetes Care 28

McCaleb, R., & Leigh, E. (2000). The encyclopedia of popular herbs: Your complete guide to the leading medicinal plants. Roseville, CA: Prima Pub.

McClain, M. (2001). The biogeochemistry of the Amazon Basin. New York: Oxford University Press.

McCutcheon A.R., Stokes W.R., Thorson L.M., Ellis S.M., Hancock R.E.W., Towers G.H.N. Anti-mycobacterial screening of British Columbian medicinal plants. International Journal of Pharmacognosy 1997 35

McDaniel, S.; Goldman, GD (2002). "Consequences of Using Escharotic Agents as Primary Treatment for Nonmelanoma Skin Cancer". Archives of Dermatology 138

McDougall GJ, Ross HA, Ikeji M, Stewart D. 2008. Berry extracts exert different antiproliferative effects against cervical and colon cancer cells grown in vitro. Journal Agricultural Food Chem. 56

McGuffin, M. American Herbal Products Association's botanical safety handbook. American Herbal Products Association.

McKay, Diane L.; Blumberg, Jeffrey B. (2007). "A review of the bioactivity of south African herbal teas: Rooibos (Aspalathus linearis) and honeybush (Cyclopia intermedia)". Phytotherapy Research 21

McKenna, D., & Jones, K. (2011). Botanical Medicines the Desk Reference for Major Herbal Supplements. (Second ed.). New York: Routledge.

Mears, R., & Hillman, G. (2007). Wild food. London: Hodder & Stoughton.

Medeiros RM, de Figueiredo AP, Benício TM, Dantas FP, Riet-Correa F (February 2008). "Teratogenicity of Mimosa

tenuiflora seeds to pregnant rats". Toxicon 51

Medicinal Herbs Article list, How to use wild herbs, herb pictures,. (n.d.). Retrieved from http://www.altnature.com/gallery/

MedlinePlus - Health Information from the National Library of Medicine. (n.d.). Retrieved from http://www.nlm.nih.gov/medlineplus/

Mill Goetz P. "Demonstration of the psychotropic effect of mother tincture of Zizyphus jujuba" Phytotherapie 2009

Mills E et al. (2005). "Impact of African herbal medicines on antiretroviral metabolism". AIDS 19

Mills, S. (1985). The dictionary of modern herbalism: A comprehensive guide to practical herbal therapy. New York: Thorsons Pub. Group

Mills, S., & Bone, K. (2000). Principles and practice of phytotherapy: Modern herbal medicine. Edinburgh: Churchill Livingstone.

Miyase T., Yamamoto R., Ueno A.,"Phenylethanoid glycosides from Stachys officinalis" Phytochemistry 1996 43

Moerman, D. (1998). Native American ethnobotany. Portland, Or.: Timber Press.

Mondal, S.; Varma, S.; Bamola, V. D.; Naik, S. N.; Mirdha, B. R.; Padhi, M. M.; Mehta, N.; Mahapatra, S. C. (2011). "Double-blinded randomized controlled trial for immunomodulatory effects of Tulsi (Ocimum sanctum Linn.) leaf extract on healthy volunteers". Journal of Ethnopharmacology 136

Moore, M. (1990). Los Remedios: Traditional Herbal Remedies of the Southwest. Santa Fe, NM: Museum of New Mexico Press.

Mori, S.; Ishikawa, C.; Nakachi, S.; Mori, N. (2011). "Anti-adult T-cell leukemia effects of Bidens pilosa". International Journal of Oncology 38

Mosquito larvicidal activity of oleic and linoleic acids isolated from Citrullus colocynthis (Linn.) Schrad A. Abdul Rahuman, P. Venkatesan and Geetha Gopalakrishnan, Parasitology Research, 2008

Muganza, D., et al. "In vitro antiprotozoal and cytotoxic activity of 33 ethonopharmacologically selected medicinal plants from Democratic Republic of Congo." J Ethnopharmacol. 2012

Mukherjee P.K., Kumar V., Mal M., Houghton P.J. "Acorus calamus: Scientific validation of ayurvedic tradition from natural resources"Pharmaceutical Biology 2007

Muñoz V , Sauvain M , Bourdy G , et al. A search for natural bioactive compounds in Bolivia through a multidisciplinary approach: Part III. Evaluation of the antimalarial activity of plants used by Alteños Indians . J Ethnopharmacol . 2000

NDL/FNIC Food Composition Database. (n.d.). Retrieved from http://ndb.nal.usda.gov/

Naftali T., Feingelernt H., Lesin Y., Rauchwarger A., Konikoff F.M. "Ziziphus jujuba extract for the treatment of chronic idiopathic constipation: A controlled clinical trial" Digestion 2008

Nahrstedt A, Butterweck V (September 1997). "Biologically active and other chemical constituents of the herb of Hypericum perforatum L". Pharmacopsychiatry 30

Nascimento, Gislene G. F.; Locatelli, Juliana; Freitas, Paulo C.; Silva, Giuliana L. (2000). "Antibacterial activity of plant extracts and phytochemicals on antibiotic-resistant bacteria". Brazilian Journal of Microbiology 31

Nathan, P. J.; Tanner, S.; Lloyd, J.; Harrison, B.; Curran, L.; Oliver, C.; Stough, C. (2004). "Effects of a combined extract of Ginkgo biloba and Bacopa monniera on cognitive function in healthy humans". Human Psychopharmacology 19

National Agricultural Library Digital Collections. (n.d.). Retrieved from http://naldc.nal.usda.gov/naldc/home.xht ml

National Center for Complementary and Alternative Medicine

National Library of Medicine - National Institutes of Health. (n.d.). Retrieved from http://www.nlm.nih.gov/

Natural carcinogenic products, EK Weisburger – Environmental Science & Technology, 1979 – ACS Publications

Newton KM, Reed SD, LaCroix AZ, Grothaus LC, Ehrlich K, Guiltinan J (2006). "Treatment of vasomotor symptoms of menopause with black cohosh, multibotanicals, soy, hormone therapy, or placebo: a randomized trial". Annals of Internal Medicine 145

Nielsen, IL; Haren, GR; Magnussen, EL; Dragsted, LO; Rasmussen, SE (2003). "Quantification of anthocyanins in commercial black currant juices by simple high-performance liquid chromatography. Investigation of their pH stability and antioxidative potency". Journal of Agricultural and Food Chemistry 51

Nishanta Rajakaruna, Cory S. Harris and G.H.N. Towers (2002). "Antimicrobial Activity of Plants Collected from Serpentine Outcrops in Sri Lanka". Pharmaceutical Biology 40

Niwano, Y.; et al., Keita; Yoshizaki, Fumihiko; Kohno, Masahiro; Ozawa, Toshihiko (2011). "Extensive screening for herbal extracts with potent antioxidant properties". Journal of Clinical Biochemistry and Nutrition 48

Noosidum A. Excito-repellency properties of essential oils from Melaleuca leucadendron L., Litsea cubeba (Lour.) Persoon and Litsea salicifolia (Nees) on Aedes aegypti (L.) mosquitoes. J Vector Ecol. 2008

Norris, LE; Collene, AL; Asp, ML; Hsu, JC; Liu, LF; Richardson, JR; Li, D, et al. (2009 Sep). "Comparison of dietary conjugated linoleic acid with safflower oil on body composition in obese postmenopausal women with type 2 diabetes mellitus.". The American journal of clinical nutrition 90

Noureddini M., Rasta V.-R. Analgesic Effect of aqueous extract of Achillea millefolium L. on rat's formalin test. Pharmacologyonline 2008

Nuntanakorn P, Jiang B, Yang H, Cervantes-Cervantes M, Kronenberg F, Kennelly EJ (2007). "Analysis of polyphenolic compounds and radical scavenging activity of four American Actaea species". Phytochem Anal 18

Obolskiy D, Pischel I, Siriwatanametanon N, Heinrich M (2009). "Garcinia mangostana L. (mangosteen): A phytochemical and pharmacological review". Phytother Res 23

Ody, P. (2000). Complete guide to medicinal herbs (2nd American ed.). New York: Dorling Kindersley.

Ogihara, Y. (2003). Sho-saiko-to: Scientific evaluation and clinical applications. London: Taylor & Francis.

Ogra, R. K. et al.; Indian calamus (Acorus calamus L.): not a tetraploid; Current Science, Vol. 97, No. 11, 10 December 2009; Current Science Association; Bangalore

Okabe, H.; Miyahara, Y.; Yamauci, T. (1982). "Studies on the constituents of Momordica charantia L.". Chemical Pharmacology Bulletin 30

O'Neill, M. J., et al. "Plants as sources of antimalarial drugs, Part 6. Activities of Simarouba amara fruits". J. Ethnopharmacol. 1988

Online Medical Dictionary. University of Newcastle upon Tyne Centre for Cancer Education. n.d.

Ott, J. (1976). Hallucinogenic Plants of North America. Berkeley, CA: Wingbow Press.

Oyebanji (2011). "Phytochemistry and in vitro anti-oxidant activities of Stellaria media, Cajanus cajan and Tetracera potatoria methanolic extracts". Journal of Medicinal Plants Research 5

Pak K.C., Lam K.Y., Law S., Tang J.C.O."The inhibitory effect of Gleditsia sinensis on cyclooxygenase-2 expression in human esophageal squamous cell carcinoma." International Journal of Molecular Medicine. 23

Pakistan encyclopaedia planta medica: A joint research project of Hamdard Foundation Pakistan and H.E.J. Research Institute of Chemistry. (1986). Karachi: Hamdard.

Pan, JG; Xu, ZL; Ji, L (1992). "Chemical studies on essential oils from 6 Artemisia species". Zhongguo Zhong yao za zhi 17

Papoutsi Z. Kassi E. Tsiapara A. Fokialakis N. Chrousos GP. Moutsatsou P. (2005). "Evaluation of estrogenic/antiestrogenic activity of ellagic acid via the estrogen receptor subtypes ERalpha and ERbeta". Journal of Agricultural & Food Chemistry 53

Parry, E. (1921). The chemistry of essential oils and artificial perfumes, (4th ed.). London: Scott, Greenwood and Son.

Parry J, Su L, Moore J et al. (May 2006). "Chemical compositions, antioxidant capacities, and antiproliferative activities of selected fruit seed flours". J. Agric. Food Chem. 54

Patel, D. K.; Prasad S.K., Kumar R., Hemalatha S. (2012). "An overview on antidiabetic medicinal plants having insulin mimetic property". Asian Pacific Journal of Tropical Biomedicine 2

Peng, X; Zhao, Y; Liang, X; Wu, L; Cui, S; Guo, A; Wang, W (2006). "Assessing the quality of RCTs on the effect of beta-elemene, one ingredient of a Chinese herb, against malignant tumors". Contemporary clinical trials 27

Perry, Ek; Pickering, At; Wang, Ww; Houghton, P; Perry, Ns (Winter 1998). "Medicinal plants and Alzheimer's disease: Integrating ethnobotanical and contemporary scientific evidence". Journal of alternative and complementary medicine (New York, N.Y.) 4

Phillips, R., & Rix, M. (2002). The botanical garden the definitive reference with more than 2000 photographs. Buffalo, NY: Firefly Books.

Phillips, R., & Rix, M. (2002). The botanical garden: Volume 1 [trees and shrubs]. London: Macmillan. Phillips / Rix

Phillips, R., & Rix, M. (2002). The botanical garden: Volume 2, [perennials and annuals]. London: Macmillan. Phillips / Rix

Physicians' desk reference 2011 (65th ed.). (2010). Montvale, N.J.: Physicians' Desk Reference.

Piacente, S; Carbone, V., Plaza, A., Zampelli, A. & Pizza, C. (2002). "Investigation of the Tuber Constituents of Maca (Lepidium meyenii Walp.)". Journal of Agricultural and Food Chemistry 50

Plant Guide. United States Department of Agriculture Natural Resources Conservation Service. May 30, 2002.

Plants, L. (2000). Proceedings of the National Seminar on the Frontiers of Research and Development in Medicinal Plants: September 16-18, 2000. Lucknow, India: Central Institute of Medicinal and Aromatic Plants.

Platt R (2000). "Current concepts in optimum nutrition for cardiovascular disease". Prev Cardiol 3

Plotkin MJ, Balick MJ (Apr 1984). "Medicinal uses of South American palms". J Ethnopharmacol 10

Polyphenolic Constituents of Fruit Pulp of Euterpe oleracea Mart. (Açai palm). S. Gallori, A. R. Bilia, M. C. Bergonzi, W. L. R. Barbosa and F. F. Vincieri, Chromatographia, 2004

Popovici M., Pârvu A.E., Oniga I., Toiu A., Tàmaş M., Benedec D. Effects of two Achillea species tinctures on experimental acute inflammation. Farmacia 2008

Potrich F.B., Allemand A., da Silva L.M., dos Santos A.C., Baggio C.H., Freitas C.S., Mendes D.A.G.B., Andre E., de Paula Werner M.F., Marques M.C.A. Antiulcerogenic activity of hydroalcoholic extract of Achillea millefolium L.: Involvement of the antioxidant system. Journal of Ethnopharmacology 2010

Pownall TL, Udenigwe CC, Aluko RE (2010). "Amino acid composition and antioxidant properties of pea seed (Pisum sativum L.) enzymatic protein hydrolysate fractions". Journal of Agricultural and Food Chemistry

Prager N, Bickett K, French N,Marcovici G (2002). "A randomized, double-blind, placebo-controlled trial to determine the effectiveness of botanically derived inhibitors of 5-a-reductase in the treatment of androgenetic alopecia". J Altern Complement Ther 8

Prakash, P.; Gupta, N. (April 2005). "Therapeutic uses of Ocimum sanctum Linn (Tulasi) with a note on eugenol and its pharmacological actions: A short review". Indian Journal of Physiology and Pharmacology 49

Premila, M. (2006). Ayurvedic herbs: A clinical guide to the healing plants of traditional Indian medicine. New York: Haworth Press.

Qiao, C.-Y., Jin-Hua Ran, Yan Li and Xiao-Quan Wang (2007): Phylogeny and Biogeography of Cedrus (Pinaceae) Inferred from Sequences of Seven Paternal Chloroplast and Maternal Mitochondrial DNA Regions. Annals of Botany

Qingdi Q. Li, Gangduo Wang, Manchao Zhang, Christopher F. Cuff, Lan Huang, Eddie Reed (2009). "β-Elemene, a novel plant-derived antineoplastic agent, increases cisplatin chemosensitivity of lung tumor cells by triggering apoptosis". Oncology Reports 22

Qiu SX, Dan C, Ding LS, Peng S, Chen SN, Farnsworth NR, Nolta J, Gross ML, Zhou P (2007). "A triterpene glycoside from black cohosh that inhibits osteoclastogenesis by modulating RANKL and TNFα signaling pathways". Chemistry & Biology 14

Rabbani GH, Butler T, Knight J, Sanyal SC, Alam K (May 1987). "Randomized controlled trial of berberine sulfate therapy for diarrhea due to enterotoxigenic Escherichia coli and Vibrio cholerae". The Journal of Infectious Diseases 155

Rai, V.; Mani, U.V.; Iyer, U.M. (1997). "Effect of Ocimum sanctum Leaf Powder on Blood Lipoproteins, Glycated Proteins and Total Amino Acids in Patients with Non-insulin-dependent Diabetes Mellitus". Journal of Nutritional and Environmental Medicine 7

Randløv C, Mehlsen J, Thomsen CF, Hedman C, von Fircks H, Winther K (March 2006). "The efficacy of St. John's Wort in patients with minor depressive symptoms or dysthymia—a double-blind placebo-controlled study". Phytomedicine 13

Rani, S.; Khan, S.A.; Ali, M. (2010). "Phytochemical investigation of the seeds of Althea officinalis L". Natural Product Research 24

Rastogi, R. (1990). Compendium of Indian medicinal plants. Lucknow: Central Drug Ray RB, Raychoudhuri A, Steele R, Nerurkar P., Bitter Melon (Momordica charantia) Extract Inhibits Breast Cancer Cell Proliferation by Modulating Cell Cycle Regulatory Genes and Promotes Apoptosis. Cancer Res. 2010

Rehder, A. 1940, reprinted 1977. Manual of cultivated trees and shrubs hardy in North America exclusive of the subtropical and warmer temperate regions. Macmillan publishing Co., Inc, New York.

Research Institute and Publications & Information Directorate, New Delhi.

Reutera, J.; C. Huykea, H. Scheuvensa, M. Plochc, K. Neumannd, T. Jakobb, C. M. Schemppa (2008). "Skin tolerance of a new bath oil containing St. John's wort extract". Skin pharmacology and physiology 21 Rahman, S., et al. "Anti-tuberculosis activity of quassinoids." Chemical Pharmacology Bulletin. 1997.

Rhoads, Ann F., Timothy A. Block, and Anna Anisko (Illustrator). The Plants of Pennsylvania: An Illustrated Manual, Second edition (2007). University of Pennsylvania Press.

Riddle, John M. (1999). Eve's Herbs: A History of Contraception and Abortion in the West. Harvard University Press.

Riehemann, K; Behnke, B; Schulze-Osthoff, K (1999). "Plant extracts from stinging nettle (Urtica dioica), an antirheumatic remedy, inhibit the proinflammatory transcription factor NF-kappaB". FEBS letters 442

Rinaldi, S. Silva, D. O. Bello, F. Alviano, C S. Alviano, D S. Matheus, ME. Fernandes, P D. (2009). Characterization of the antinociceptive and anti-inflammatory activities from Cocos nucifera L. (Palmae). Journal of Ethnopharmacology 122

Ritchie, F. (1999). Handbook of edible wild plants and weeds. Springfield, Or.: Ritchie Unlimited Publications.

Rivera-Arce E, Chávez-Soto MA, Herrera-Arellano A et al. (February 2007). "Therapeutic effectiveness of a Mimosa tenuiflora cortex extract in venous leg ulceration treatment". J Ethnopharmacol 109

Rivera-Arce E, Gattuso M, Alvarado R et al. (September 2007). "Pharmacognostical studies of the plant drug Mimosae tenuiflorae cortex". J Ethnopharmacol 113

Rodrigues, Eliana & Carlini, E.A. (2006): Plants with possible psychoactive effects used by the Krahô Indians, Brazil. Revista Brasileira de Psiquiatria

Roodenrys, S.; Booth, D.; Bulzomi, S.; Phipps, A.; Micallef, C.; Smoker, J. (2002). "Chronic effects of Brahmi (Bacopa monnieri) on human memory". Neuropsychopharmacology 27

Rose, J. (1987). Jeanne Rose's modern herbal. New York, N.Y.: Perigee Books.

Rosengarten, Frederic, Jr. (2004). The Book of Edible Nuts. Dover Publications.

Ross, I. (1999). Medicinal plants of the world: Chemical constituents, traditional, and modern medicinal uses. Totowa, N.J.: Humana Press.

Ross, J. (2003). Combining Western herbs and Chinese medicine: Principles, practice, and materia medica. Seattle, Wash.: Greenfields Press.

Roy, K.; Thakur M., Dixit V.K. (2007). "Effect of Citrullus colocynthis on hair growth in albino rats". Pharmaceutical Biology 45

Royal Horticultural Society; http://apps.rhs.org.uk/plantselector/

Said, O., Khalil, K. Fulder, S. and Azaizeh, H. Ethnopharmacological Survey of the Medicinal herbs in Israel, the Golan Heights and the West Bank Region. Journal of Ethnopharmacology, 83

Sairam K. Priyambada S. Aryya NC. Goel RK.Gastroduodenal ulcer protective activity of Asparagus racemosus: an experimental, biochemical and histological study. Journal of Ethnopharmacology. 86

Sale C, Harris RC, Delves S, Corbett J (May 2006). "Metabolic and physiological effects of ingesting extracts of bitter orange, green tea and guarana at rest and during treadmill walking in overweight males". Int J Obes (Lond) 30

Salunkhe, D.K., J.K. Chavan, R.N. Adsule, and S.S. Kadam. (1992). World Oilseeds – Chemistry, Technology, and Utilization. Springer.

Samorini, Giorgio (2002). Animals and psychedelics: the natural world and the instinct to alter consciousness.

Sayyah, M.; Saroukhani, G.; Peirovi, A.; Kamalinejad, M. (August 2003). "Analgesic and anti-inflammatory activity of the leaf essential oil of Laurus nobilis Linn". Phytother Res 17

Schafferman, D.; Beharav A., Shabelsky E., Yaniv Z (1998). "Evaluation of Citrullus colocynthis, a desert plant native in Israel, as a potential source of edible oil". Journal of Arid Environments 40

Schauss A.G., Wu X., Prior R.L., Ou B., Huang D., Owens J., Agarwal A., Jensen G.S., Hart A.N., Shanbrom E. (2006). "Antioxidant capacity and other bioactivities of the freeze-dried amazonian palm berry, Euterpe oleraceae Mart. (acai)". J Agric Food Chem 54

Schnitzler, P; Schuhmacher, A; Astani, A; Reichling, J (2008). "Melissa officinalis oil affects infectivity of enveloped herpesviruses". Phytomedicine 15

Scholey, A B (2003). "Modulation of Mood and Cognitive Performance Following Acute Administration of Single Doses of Melissa Officinalis (Lemon Balm) with Human CNS Nicotinic and Muscarinic Receptor-Binding Properties". Neuropsychopharmacology 28

Schubert SY, Lansky EP, Neeman I (July, 1999). "Antioxidant and eicosanoid enzyme inhibition properties of pomegranate seed oil and fermented juice flavonoids". J Ethnopharmacol 66

Schultz, Gretchen; Peterson, Chris; Coats, Joel (2006). "Natural Insect Repellents: Activity against Mosquitoes and Cockroaches"

Schulz, V. (2004). Rational phytotherapy: A reference guide for physicians and pharmacists (5th ed.). Berlin: Springer.

Seal S, Chatterjee P, Bhattacharya S, Pal D, Dasgupta S, et al. (2012) Vapor of Volatile Oils from Litsea cubeba Seed Induces Apoptosis and Causes Cell Cycle Arrest in Lung Cancer Cells. PLoS ONE 7

Seden K. Dickinson L. Khoo S. Back D.. Grapefruit-drug interactions. [Review]. Drugs. 2010. 70.

Sheeja K, Shihab PK, Kuttan G. Antioxidant and inflammatory modulating activities of the plant Andrographis paniculata Nees, Immunopharmacol Immunotoxicol. 2006.

Seeram NP, Aronson WJ, Zhang Y et al. (September 2007). "Pomegranate ellagitannin-derived metabolites inhibit prostate cancer growth and localize to the mouse prostate gland". J. Agric. Food Chem. 55

Semiz, A, Sen A. (February 2007). "Antioxidant and chemoprotective properties of Momordica charantia L. (bitter melon) fruit extract". African Journal of Biotechnology 6

Seeram, NP (2008). "Berry fruits: compositional elements, biochemical activities, and the impact of their intake on human health, performance, and disease". Journal of Agricultural and Food Chemistry 56

Seidl, P. (1995). Chemistry of the Amazon: Biodiversity, natural products, and environmental issues : Developed from the First International Symosium on Chemistry and the Amazon sponsored by the Associação Brasileira de Química, American Chemical Semiz, A, Sen A. (February 2007). "Antioxidant and chemoprotective properties of Momordica charantia L. (bitter melon) fruit extract". African Journal of Biotechnology 6

Seo SW et al. (Jan 2011). "Protective effects of Curcuma longa against cerulein-induced acute pancreatitis and pancreatitis-associated lung injury". Int J Mol Med 27

Sharma K. Bhatnagar M. Kulkarni SK. "Effect of Convolvulus pluricaulis Choisy and Asparagus racemosus Willd on learning and memory in young and old

mice: a comparative evaluation." Indian Journal of Experimental Biology. 48

Sharma, P.; Kulshreshtha, S.; Sharma, A.L. (1998). "Anti-cataract activity of Ocimum sanctum on experimental cataract". Indian Journal of Pharmacology 30

Sharma U. Saini R. Kumar N. Singh B. Steroidal saponins from Asparagus racemosus. Chemical & Pharmaceutical Bulletin. 57

Shi J, Yu J, Pohorly JE, Kakuda Y (2003). "Polyphenolics in grape seeds-biochemistry and functionality". Journal Medicinal Food 6

Shibib, BA; Khan, LA; Rahman, R (May 15). "Hypoglycemic activity of Coccinia indica and Momordica charantia in diabetic rats: depression of the hepatic gluconeogenic enzymes glucose-6-phosphatase and fructose-1,6-bisphosphatase and elevation of both liver and red-cell shunt enzyme glucose-6-phosphate dehydrogenase". Biochem J. 292

Shin HR, Kim JY, Yun TK, Morgan G, Vainio H (2000). "The cancer-preventive potential of Panax ginseng: a review of human and experimental evidence". Cancer Causes Control 11

Shukla, A.; Rasik, A. M.; Jain, G. K.; Shankar, R.; Kulshrestha, D. K.; Dhawan, B. N. (1999). "In vitro and in vivo wound healing activity of asiaticoside isolated from Centella asiatica". Journal of Ethnopharmacology 65

Shukla PK, Khanna VK, Ali MM, Maurya R, Khan MY, Srimal RC. "Neuroprotective effect of Acorus calamus against middle cerebral artery occlusion-induced ischaemia in rat" Hum Exp Toxicology 2006.

Silva FL, Fischer DC, Tavares JF, Silva MS, de Athayde-Filho PF, Barbosa-Filho JM.,"Compilation of secondary metabolites from Bidens pilosa L." Molecules, 2011

Simic, M; Kundaković, T; Kovacević, N (September 2003). "Preliminary assay on the antioxidative activity of Laurus nobilis extracts". Fitoterapia 74

Simon PW (1997). Plant Pigments for Color and Nutrition.

Singh, A.; Singh, S. K. (2009). "Evaluation of antifertility potential of Brahmi in male mouse". Contraception 79

Singh GK. Garabadu D. Muruganandam AV. Joshi VK. Krishnamurthy S. Antidepressant activity of Asparagus racemosus in rodent models. Pharmacology, Biochemistry & Behavior. 91

Sinisalo, Marjatta; Enkovaara, Anna-Liisa; Kivistö, Kari T. (2010). "Possible hepatotoxic effect of rooibos tea: A case report". European Journal of Clinical Pharmacology 66

Small, E., & Catling, P. (1999). Canadian medicinal crops. Ottawa: NRC Research Press.

Society, Centro de Tecnologia Mineral, and Instituto Nacional de Pesquisas da Amazonia Manaus, Amazonas, Brazil, November 21-25, 1993. Washington, DC: Smith, A, (1997). A Gardener's Handbook of Plant Names: Their Meanings and Origins. Dover Publications

Smith, P; MacLennan, K; Darlington, CL (1996). "The neuroprotective properties of the Ginkgo biloba leaf: a review of the possible relationship to platelet-activating factor (PAF)". Journal of Ethnopharmacology 50

Stuart, M. (1981). The Encyclopedia of herbs and herbalism. New York: Crescent Books

South, G., & Whittick, A. (1987). Introduction to phycology. Oxford [Oxfordshire: Blackwell Scientific Publications.

Stablein JJ. Melaleuca tree and respiratory disease. Ann Allergy Asthma Immunol. 2002

Standley, L; Winterton, P; Marnewick, JL; Gelderblom, WC; Joubert, E; Britz, TJ (2001 Jan). "Influence of processing stages on antimutagenic and antioxidant potentials of rooibos tea.". Journal of Agricultural and Food Chemistry 49

Stough, C.; Downey, L. A.; Lloyd, J.; Silber, B.; Redman, S.; Hutchison, C.; Wesnes, K.; Nathan, P. J. (2008). "Examining the nootropic effects of a special extract of Bacopa Monniera on human cognitive functioning: 90 day double-blind placebo-controlled randomized trial". Phytotherapy Research 22

Streloke, M. et al.; Ascher, K. R. S.; Schmidt, G. H.; Neumann, W. P. (1989). "Vapor pressure and volatility of β-asarone, the main ingredient of an indigenous stored-product insecticide, Acorus calamus oil". Phytoparasitica 17

Sturtevant, WC (1955). The Mikasuki Seminole: Medical Beliefs and Practices. Ann Arbor, MI: University Microfilms.

Stuttgart: Georg Thieme Verlag. Biology and chemistry of active natural substances: International symposium, Bonn, July 17-22, 1990, plenary lectures. (1991).

Suanarunsawat, T.; Boonnak, T.; Na Ayutthaya, W. D.; Thirawarapan, S. (2010). "Anti-hyperlipidemic and cardioprotective effects of Ocimum sanctum L. fixed oil in rats fed a high fat diet". Journal of Basic and Clinical Physiology and Pharmacology 21

Suh SO, Kroh M, Kim NR, Joh YG, Cho MY. (2002). "Effects of red ginseng upon postoperative immunity and survival in patients with stage III gastric cancer". American Journal of Chinese Medicine. 30

Sultan S, Spector J, Mitchell RM (December 2006). "Ischemic colitis associated with use of a bitter orange-containing dietary weight-loss supplement". Mayo Clinic Proceedings 81

Sun, Meng; Lou, Wei; Chun, Jae Yeon; Cho, Daniel S.; Nadiminty, Nagalakshmi; Evans, Christopher P. et al. (2010). "Sanguinarine Suppresses Prostate Tumor Growth and Inhibits Survivin Expression". Genes & Cancer 1

Szapary, PO; Wolfe, ML; Bloedon, LT; Cucchiara, AJ; Dermarderosian, AH; Cirigliano, MD; Rader, DJ (2003). "Guggulipid Ineffective for Lowering Cholesterol". JAMA 290

T. Ogasawara, k.Chiba, m.Tada in (Y. P. S. Bajaj ed). 1988. Medicinal and Aromatic Plants, Volume 10. Springer,

Taati, Majid; Masoud Alirezaei, Mohamad Hadi Moshkatalsadat, Bahram Rasoulian, Mehrnoush Moghadasi, Farzam Sheikhzadeh, Ali Sokhtezari. (2011). "Protective effects of Ziziphus jujuba fruit extract against ethanol-induced hippocampal oxidative stress and spatial memory impairment in rats". Journal of Medicinal Plants Research 5

Tan, NH; Fung, SY; Sim, SM; Marinello, E; Guerranti, R; Aguiyi, JC (2009). "The protective effect of Mucuna pruriens seeds against snake venom poisoning". Journal of Ethnopharmacology 123

Tanacetum Balsamita L: A Medicinal Plant. M.J. Pérez-Alonso, A. Velasco-Negueruela, A. Burzaco

Tang J., Wang C.K., Pan X., Yan H., Zeng G., Xu W., He W., Daly N.L., Craik D.J., Tan N."Isolation and characterization of cytotoxic cyclotides from Viola tricolor" Peptides 2010

Tang SY, Gruber J, Wong KP, Halliwell B (April 2007). "Psoralea corylifolia L. inhibits mitochondrial complex I and proteasome activities in SH-SY5Y cells". Ann. N. Y. Acad. Sci. 1100: 486–96.

Tang W.K., Chui C.H., Fatima S., Kok S.H., Pak K.C., Ou T.M., Hui K.S., Wong M.M., Wong J., Law S., Tsao S.W., Lam K.Y., Beh P.S., Srivastava G., Ho K.P., Chan A.S., Tang J.C. "Inhibitory effects of Gleditsia sinensis fruit extract on telomerase activity and oncogenic

expression in human esophageal squamous cell carcinoma." International journal of molecular medicine. 19. 2007.

Tannin-Spitz, T.; Grossman S., Dovrat S., Gottlieb H.E., Bergman M. (2007). "Growth inhibitory activity of cucurbitacin glucosides isolated from Citrullus colocynthis on human breast cancer cells". Biochemical Pharmacology 73

Tatsis, EC; Boeren, S; Exarchou, V; Troganis, AN; Vervoort, J; Gerothanassis, IP (2007). "Identification of the major constituents of Hypericum perforatum by LC/SPE/NMR and/or LC/MS". Phytochemistry 68

Taur D.J., Patil R.Y.,"Mast cell stabilizing, antianaphylactic and antihistaminic activity of Coccinia grandis fruits in asthma". Chinese Journal of Natural Medicines. 9

Taylor, Frederick R. (2011). "Nutraceuticals and Headache: The Biological Basis". Headache: the Journal of Head and Face Pain 51

Taylor LG (2005). The healing power of rainforest herbs: a guide to understanding and using herbal medicinals. Garden City Park, NY: Square One Publishers.

Teschke, R; Bahre, R (2009). "Severe hepatotoxicity by Indian Ayurvedic herbal products: A structured causality assessment". Annals of hepatology 8.

Teucher, T; Obertreis, B; Ruttkowski, T; Schmitz, H (1996). "Cytokine secretion in whole blood of healthy subjects following oral administration of Urtica dioica L. Plant extract". Arzneimittel-Forschung 46

Thakur M. Chauhan NS. Bhargava S. Dixit VK. A comparative study on aphrodisiac activity of some ayurvedic herbs in male albino rats. Archives of Sexual Behavior. 38

The Organic Gardener's Handbook of Natural Pest and Disease, Fern Marshall Bradley, Barbara W. Ellis, Deborah L. Martin,

The pharmacopœia of the United States of America: (the United States pharmacopœia). (12th revision (U.S.P. XII) / ed.). (1942). Washington, D.C.: Published by the Board of Trustees

The Pharmacopoeia of the United States of America (The United States pharmacopoeia) 19th rev. (1974). Rockville, Md.: United States Pharmacopeial Convention.

The use of herbal medicines by people with cancer: A qualitative study. (2009). BioMed Central.

"Therapeutic effect of arctiin and arctigenin in immunocompetent and immunocompromised mice infected with

influenza" Biological and Pharmaceutical Bulletin 2010

Thierer, John W., Niering, William A., and Olmstead, Nancy C. (2001) National Audubon Society Field Guide to North American Wildflowers, Eastern Region, Revised Edition. Alfred A. Knopf

Thompson LU, Chen JM, Li T, Strasser-Weippl K, Goss PE (2005). "Dietary flaxseed alters tumor biological markers in postmenopausal breast cancer". Clinical Cancer Research 11

Thomson, W. (1978). Healing Plants: A modern herbal. London: Macmillan.

Tipton, K. (1979). Neurochemistry and biochemical pharmacology. Baltimore: University Park Press.

Tiwari M, Dwivedi UN, Kakkar P. 2010. Suppression of oxidative stress and pro-inflammatory mediators by Cymbopogon citratus D. Stapf extract in lipopolysaccharide stimulated murine alveolar macrophages. Food Chemistry Toxicology

Toiu A. Muntean E. Oniga I. Vostinaru O. Tamas M. " Pharmacognostic research on Viola tricolor L. (Violaceae)." Revista Medico-Chirurgicala a Societatii de Medici Si Naturalisti Din Iasi. 1

Toiu A. Parvu AE. Oniga I. Tamas M."Evaluation of anti-inflammatory activity of alcoholic extract from Viola tricolor.", Revista Medico-Chirurgicala a Societatii de Medici Si Naturalisti Din Iasi. 11

Trease, G. (1952). A Text-Book of Pharmacognosy ... Sixth edition. Pp. viii. 821. Baillière, Tindall & Cox: London.

Tsch, C. (2005). The encyclopedia of psychoactive plants: Ethnopharmacology and its applications. Rochester, Vt.: Park Street Press.

Tsuda H; Ohshima Y; Nomoto H et al. (2004). "Cancer prevention by natural compounds". Drug Metabolism and Pharmacokinetics 19

Tulyaganov, T. S.; Nigmatullaev, A. M. (2000). Chemistry of Natural Compounds 36

Tutin, T. (1976). Flora Europaea. Cambridge: Cambridge University Press.

Ukiya M, Akihisa T, Yasukawa K et al. Anti-inflammatory, anti-tumor-promoting, and cytotoxic activities of constituents of pot marigold (Calendula officinalis) flowers. (2006).

Umek, A; Kreft, S; Kartnig, T; Heydel, B (1999). "Quantitative phytochemical analyses of six hypericum species growing in slovenia". Planta medica 65

UN Food & Agriculture Organisation | Online references | cyclopaedia.net. (n.d.). Retrieved from http://www.cyclopaedia.info/UN-Food-and-Agriculture-Organisation

Valdes, A., et al. "In vitro anti-microbial activity of the Cuban medicinal plants Simarouba glauca DC, Melaleuca leucadendron L and Artemisia absinthium L." Mem Inst Oswaldo Cruz. 2008

Valeriote, F. A., et al. "Anticancer activity of glaucarubinone analogues." Oncol Res. 1998

Vaughan, J.G.; Geissler, C.A. (1997). The New Oxford Book of Food Plants. Oxford University Press.

Veronese ML, Gillen LP, Burke JP, Dorval EP, Hauck WW, Pequignot E, Waldman SA, Greenberg HE. Exposure-dependent inhibition of intestinal and hepatic CYP3A4 in vivo by grapefruit juice. Journal of Clinical Pharmacology. 2003;43

Visarata, N.; Ungsurungsie, M. (1981). "Extracts from Momordica charantiaL". Pharmaceutical Biology 19

Volz, S. M., and S. S. Renner (Volz and Renner) 2009. Phylogeography of the ancient Eurasian medicinal plant genus Bryonia (Cucurbitaceae) inferred from nuclear and chloroplast sequences. Taxon 58

von Woedtke T, Schlüter B, Pflegel P, Lindequist U, Jülich WD (June 1999). "Aspects of the antimicrobial efficacy of grapefruit seed extract and its relation to preservative substances contained". Pharmazie 54

Vukics V. Kery A. Guttman A."Analysis of polar antioxidants in Heartsease (Viola tricolor L.) and Garden pansy (Viola x wittrockiana Gams.)". Journal of Chromatographic Science. 46

Waako PJ, Gumede B, Smith P, Folb PI (May 2005). "The in vitro and in vivo antimalarial activity of Cardiospermum halicacabum L. and Momordica foetida Schumch. Et Thonn". J Ethnopharmacol 99

Wada L, Ou B (June 2002). "Antioxidant activity and phenolic content of Oregon caneberries". Journal of Agricultural and Food Chemistry 50

Wagh S., Vidhale N.N. (2010). "Antimicrobial efficacy of Boerhaavia diffusa against some human pathogenic bacteria and fungi". Biosciences Biotechnology Research Asia 7

Wagner, Hildebert (1999). Immunomodulatory agents from plants. Birkhäuser.

Wang C., Xia Y.F., Gao Z.Z., Lu D., Dai Y. "Inhibition of mast cell degranulation by saponins from Gleditsia sinensis-structure-activity relationships." Natural Product Communications. 4. 2009

Wang JJ, Shi QH, Zhang W, Sanderson BJ (2012). "Anti-skin cancer properties from phenolic-rich extract from the pericarp of mangosteen (Garcinia mangostana Linn.)". Food Chemistry Toxicology 50

Wang, Lu et al. (2009). "Ultrasonic nebulization extraction coupled with headspace single drop microextraction and gas chromatography–mass spectrometry for analysis of the essential oil in Cuminum cyminum L". Analytica Chimica Acta 647

Wang ZT, Ng TB, Yeung HW, Xu GJ (December 1996). "Immunomodulatory effect of a polysaccharide-enriched preparation of Codonopsis pilosula roots". Gen. Pharmacol. 27 Warrier, P. K.; V. P. K. Nambiar, C. Ramankutty, R. Vasudevan Nair (1996). Indian medicinal plants. Orient Blackswan.

Weber HA, Zart MK, Hodges AE, et al. (December 2003). "Chemical comparison of goldenseal (Hydrastis canadensis L.) root powder from three commercial suppliers". Journal of Agricultural and Food Chemistry 51 Weber W, Vander Stoep A, McCarty RL, Weiss NS, Biederman J, McClellan J (June 2008). "A Randomized Placebo Controlled Trial Of Hypericum perforatum For Attention Deficit Hyperactivity Disorder In Children And Adolescents". JAMA 299

Webster, D.E.; J. Lu, S.-N. Chen, N.R. Farnsworth and Z. Jim Wang (2006). "Activation of the μ-opiate receptor by Vitex agnus-castus methanol extracts: Implication for its use in PMS". Journal of Ethnopharmacology 106

Weerasinghe, Priya; Hallock, Sarathi; Brown, Robert E.; Loose, David S.; Buja, L. Maximilian (2012). "A model for cardiomyocyte cell death: Insights into mechanisms of oncosis". Experimental and Molecular Pathology.

Weinmann, S; Roll, S; Schwarzbach, C; Vauth, C; Willich, SN (2010). "Effects of Ginkgo biloba in dementia: systematic review and meta-analysis". BMC geriatrics 10

Weisskopf. Schaffner. Jundt. Sulser. Wyler. Tullberg-Reinert. Planta Medica 2005

Wells, A., Edwards, E.D., Houston, W. W. K., Lepidoptera: Hesperioidea, Papilionoidea, Volume 31, CSIRO, 2001.

Wheatley D (2004). "Triple-blind, placebo-controlled trial of Ginkgo biloba in sexual dysfunction due to antidepressant drugs". Hum Psychopharmacol 19.

Wilt TJ, Ishani A, Rutks I, MacDonald R (2000). "Phytotherapy for benign prostatic hyperplasia". Public Health Nutr 3

Winston, David & Maimes, Steven. "Adaptogens: Herbs for Strength, Stamina, and Stress Relief," Healing Arts Press, 2007.

Whitford AC (1941). "Textile fibers used in eastern aboriginal North America". Anthropological Papers of the American Museum of Natural History 38

Wichtl, Max,Herbal drugs and phytopharmaceuticals: a handbook,2004

Wild Medicinal Plants: What to Look For, When to Harvest, How to Use 2002 Schneider / Mellichamp

William Thomas Fernie, Herbal Simples Approved for Modern Uses of Cure, 3rd enlarged ed. Bristol: Wright, 1914

Williamson, E. (2009). Stockley's herbal medicines interactions a guide to the interactions of herbal medicines, dietary supplements and nutraceuticals with conventional medicines. London: Pharmaceutical Press.

Wilt T, Ishani A, Mac Donald R (2002). "Serenoa repens for benign prostatic hyperplasia". In Tacklind, James. Cochrane Database Syst Rev (3): CD001423.

Winston & Kuhn's Herbal Therapy & Supplements: A Scientific and Traditional Approach 2007 Kuhn / Winston

Witkowska-Banaszczak E., Bylka W., Matławska I., Goślińska O., Muszyński Z. ,"Antimicrobial activity of Viola tricolor herb". Fitoterapia 2005

Wong AHC, Smith M, Boon HS (1998). "Herbal remedies in psychiatric practice". Arch Gen Psychiatry 55

Wright CI, Van-Buren L, Kroner CI, Koning MM (October 2007). "Herbal medicines as diuretics: a review of the scientific evidence". J Ethnopharmacol 114

Wright SC. Maree JE. Sibanyoni M. Treatment of oral thrush in HIV/AIDS patients with lemon juice and lemon grass (Cymbopogon citratus) and gentian violet. Phytomedicine. 16. 2009.

Wyk, B., & Wink, M. (2004). Medicinal plants of the world: An illustrated scientific guide to important medicinal plants and their uses. Portland: Timber Press.

Xie L.-H., Ahn E.-M., Akao T., Abdel-Hafez A.A.-M., Nakamura N., Hattori M."Transformation of arctiin to estrogenic and antiestrogenic substances by human intestinal bacteria" Chemical and Pharmaceutical Bulletin 2003

Xu XM, Li L, Chen M., "Studies on the chemical constituents of Schisandra pubescens". Zhong Yao Cai. 2009

Xu Y.J., Han C.J., Xu S.J., Yu X., Jiang G.Z., Nan C.H. "Effects of Acanthopanax senticosus on learning and memory in a mouse model of Alzheimer's disease and protection against free radical injury to brain tissue" Neural Regeneration Research 2008

Yamada, K.; Hung, P.; Park, T. K.; Park, P. J.; Limb, B. O. (2011). "A comparison of the immunostimulatory effects of the medicinal herbs Echinacea, Ashwagandha and Brahmi". Journal of Ethnopharmacology 137

Yemm RS, Poulton JE (June 1986). "Isolation and characterization of multiple forms of mandelonitrile lyase from mature black cherry (Prunus serotina Ehrh.) seeds". Archives of biochemistry and biophysics 247

Yeung, H. (1985). Handbook of Chinese herbs and formulas. Los Angeles, U.S.A.: H.C. Yeung.

Yeung. Him-Che. Handbook of Chinese Herbs and Formulas. 1985. Los Angeles: Institute of Chinese Medicine.

Yoo, Ki-Yeon; Hua Li, In Koo Hwang, Jung Hoon Choi, Choong Hyun Lee, Dae Young Kwon, Shi Yong Ryu, Young Sup Kim, Il-Jun Kang, Hyung-Cheul Shin, and Moo-Ho Won. (2010). "Zizyphus Attenuates Ischemic Damage in the Gerbil Hippocampus via Its Antioxidant Effect". Journal of Medicinal Food 13

Yoshikawa M, Murakami T, Kishi A et al. (2001). Medicinal flowers. III. Marigold.(1): hypoglycemic, gastric emptying inhibitory, and gastroprotective principles and new oleanane-type triterpene oligolycosides, calendasaponins A, B, C, and D, from Egyptian Calendula officinalis. Chem Pharm

Yu, Xiuzhu; Van De Voort, Frederick R.; Li, Zhixi; Yue, Tianli (2007). "Proximate Composition of the Apple Seed and Characterization of Its Oil". International Journal of Food Engineering 3

Yuan CS, Mehendale S, Xiao Y, Aung HH, Xie JT, Ang-Lee MK (2004). "The gamma-aminobutyric acidergic effects of valerian and valerenic acid on rat brainstem neuronal activity.". Anesth Analg 98

Yun TK, Lee YS, Lee YH, Kim SI, Yun HY (2001). "Anticarcinogenic effect of Panax ginseng C.A. Meyer and identification of active compounds". Journal of Korean Medical Science 16

Zakay-Rones, Zichria; Noemi Varsano, Moshe Zlotnik, Orly Manor, Liora Regev, Miriam Schlesinger, Madeleine Mumcuoglu (1995). "Inhibition of Several Strains of Influenza Virus in Vitro and Reduction of Symptoms by an Elderberry Extract (Sambucus nigra L.) during an Outbreak of Influenza B Panama" (PDF). J Altern Complement Med 1

Zakim, D. (1985). Biochemical pharmacology and toxicology. New York: Wiley. Biochemical Pharmacology. 2011

Zarse, K., et al. "The phytochemical glaucarubinone promotes mitochondrial metabolism, reduces body fat, and extends lifespan of Caenorhabditis elegans." Horm Metab Res. 2011

Zhang XW, Li WF, Li WW, Ren KH, Fan CM, Chen YY, Shen YL (2011). "Protective effects of the aqueous extract of Scutellaria baicalensis against acrolein-induced oxidative stress in cultured

human umbilical vein endothelial cells". Pharm Biol 49

Zhao F., Wang L., Liu K. "In vitro anti-inflammatory effects of arctigenin, a lignan from Arctium lappa L., through inhibition on iNOS pathway" Journal of Ethnopharmacology 2009

Zhao G, Li S, Qin GW, Fei J, Guo LH (2007). "Inhibitive effects of Fructus Psoraleae extract on dopamine transporter and noradrenaline transporter.". J Ethnopharmacol 112 (3): 498–506.

Zhou L., Li D., Wang J., Liu Y., Wu J."Antibacterial phenolic compounds from the spines of Gleditsia sinensis Lam." Natural Product Research. 21. 2007.

Zhao LH, Huang CY, Shan Z, Xiang BG, Mei LH (2005). "Fingerprint analysis of Psoralea corylifolia by HLPC and LC-MS". J Chromatogr B 821: 67–74.

Zhu X. Zhang W. Zhao J. Wang J. Qu W. Hypolipidaemic and hepatoprotective effects of ethanolic and aqueous extracts from Asparagus officinalis L. by-products in mice fed a high-fat diet. Journal of the Science of Food & Agriculture. 90

Zick S.M., Sen A., Feng Y., Green J., Olatunde S., Boon H."Trial of essiac to ascertain its effect in women with breast cancer (TEA-BC)" Journal of Alternative and Complementary Medicine 2006

Zillur Rahman and M. Shamim Jairajpuri. Neem in Unani Medicine. Neem Research and Development Society of Pesticide Science, India, New Delhi, 1993. Edited by N.S. Randhawa and B.S. Parmar. 2nd revised edition

Spencer, C. F., et al. "Survey of plants for antimalarial activity." Lloydia 1947

Index

188